International travel and health

Situation as on 1 January 2002

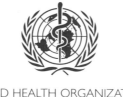

WORLD HEALTH ORGANIZATION
GENEVA
2002

The information given in this publication is valid on the date of issue. It should be kept up to date with the notes of amendments published in the *Weekly epidemiological record* (http://www.who.int/wer).

Any comments or questions concerning this publication should be addressed to:

Information Resource Centre
Communicable Diseases
World Health Organization
1211 Geneva 27, Switzerland
fax: (+41) 22 791 4285
email: cdsdoc@who.int

World Wide Web access: http://www.who.int/ith

WHO Library Cataloguing-in-Publication Data

International travel and health: situation as on 1 January 2002.

1. Communicable disease control   2. Travel   3. Vaccination

ISBN 92 4 158027 5   (NLM Classification: WA 110)
ISSN 0254-296X

Designed by minimum graphics
Cover designed by WHO/CDS and Calliscope
Cover photos: Market scene, Bolivia: WHO/PAHO/A. Waak
          Crowd scene, Bangladesh: WHO/H. Anenden
          Village, Côte d'Ivoire: WHO/STILLS/M. Edwards
          Beach, Mozambique: W. Worwang

Printed in Switzerland
2001/14172 – ATAR – 12500

Contents

Acknowledgements

WHO gratefully acknowledges the collaboration of travel medicine experts and end-users of *International travel and health* who have provided advice and information during the preparation of this edition. The following individuals were consulted and those who made contributions are thanked:

Professor Joao Luis Baptista, Centro de Investigação em Saúde Comunitária (CISCOS), Departamento de Saúde Publica, Universidade Nova de Lisboa, Lisbon, Portugal

Dr Ron Behrens, Department of Infectious and Tropical Diseases, London School of Tropical Medicine and Hygiene, London, England

Dr Mads Buhl, Department of Infectious Diseases, Aarhus University Hospital, Aarhus, Denmark

Dr Fernando Carreras, Direccion general de salud publica y consumo, Sanidad exterior y veterinaria, Madrid, Spain

Dr Christine Chevalier, Responsable du service médical, Médecins sans Frontières (MSF), Geneva, Switzerland

Dr Claus Curdt-Christiansen, Chief, Aviation Medicine Section, International Civil Aviation Organization (ICAO), Montreal, Canada

Dr Roz Dewart, Division of Quarantine, Centers for Disease Control and Prevention (CDC), Atlanta, GA, USA

Mr Tom Frens, Managing Editor, Shoreland Inc., Milwaukee, WI, USA

Dr Tony Gherardin, Regional Medical Director for Asia, Department of Immigration and Multicultural Affairs, Australian Embassy, Bangkok, Thailand

Mr Henryk Handszuh, Chief, Quality of Tourism Development, World Tourism Organization, Madrid, Spain

Dr Jay Keystone, Professor of Medicine, University of Toronto, Tropical Disease Unit, Toronto General Hospital, Toronto, Canada

Dr Phyllis E. Kozarsky, Chief, Travelers' Health, Division of Quarantine, Centers for Disease Control and Prevention (CDC), Atlanta, GA, USA

Dr Gil Lea, Travel Medicine Unit, Communicable Diseases Surveillance Centre (CDSC), Public Health Laboratory Service, London, United Kingdom

Dr Dominique Legros, EPICENTRE, Paris, France

Dr Louis Loutan, Département de médecine communautaire, Hôpital cantonal de Genève, Geneva, Switzerland

Dr Hannah Nohynek, Project Coordinator, National Public Health Institute, Helsinki, Finland

Dr Walter Pasini, WHO Collaborating Centre for Tourist and Travel Medicine, Rimini, Italy

Dr Volker Schulte, Fondation suisse pour la promotion de la santé, Lausanne, Switzerland

Mr Richard Smithies, Director, Policy Analysis, Government and Industry Affairs, International Air Transport Association (IATA), Geneva, Switzerland

Professor Robert Steffen, Head, Division of Communicable Diseases, Institute of Social and Preventive Medicine, University of Zurich, Zurich, Switzerland

Dr Alfons Van Gompel, Head, Polyclinic–Travel Clinic, Associate Professor in Tropical Medicine, Institute of Tropical Medicine, Antwerp, Belgium

Dr Eric Walker, Head, Travel Medicine Division, Scottish Centre for Infection and Environmental Health, Glasgow, United Kingdom

Dr Jane Zuckermann, Medical Director, Academic Centre for Travel Medicine and Vaccines and Royal Free Travel Health Centre, Royal Free and University College Medical School, London, United Kingdom

The following WHO personnel made contributions in their fields of expertise:

Executive Editor: Dr Lindsay Martinez

Contributors: Dr Antero Aitio, Dr Jean-Charles Alary (retired), Dr Ray Arthur, Mrs Sarah Ballance, Dr James Bartram, Dr Daniel Bleed, Dr Robert Bos, Dr Andrea Bosman, Ms Judith Canny, Dr Claire-Lise Chaignat, Dr John Clements, Dr Philippe Desjeux, Dr Brian Doberstyn, Dr Antonio Gerbase, Dr Pascale Gilbert-Miguet, Mrs Anne Guilloux, Dr Max Hardiman, Dr Jean Jannin, Mrs Mary-Kay Kindhauser, Dr Douglas Klaucke, Dr Daniel Lavanchy, Dr Stefano Lazzari, Ms Sarah Mahon, Dr Shanthi Mendis, Dr François-Xavier Meslin, Dr Luc Noël, Dr Hitoshi Oshitani, Ms Margaret Peden, Mrs Albane Perdrix, Dr Jenny Pronczuk, Dr Michael Repacholi, Dr Maura Ricketts, Dr Aafje Rietveld, Dr Pascal Ringwald, Dr Guénaël Rodier, Dr Cathy Roth, Dr Colin Roy, Dr Lorenzo Savioli, Dr Inon Schenker, Dr Evgueni Tikhomirov, Ms Mary Vallanjon, Miss Christèle Wantz, Dr Jay Wenger, Mrs Martine White.

Preface

International travel is undertaken by large, and ever increasing, numbers of people for professional, social, recreational and humanitarian purposes. More people travel greater distances and at greater speed than ever before, and this upward trend looks set to continue. Travellers are thus exposed to a variety of health risks in unfamiliar environments. Most such risks, however, can be minimized by suitable precautions taken before, during and after travel, and it is the purpose of this book to provide guidance on measures to prevent or reduce any adverse consequences for travellers' health.

This edition of *International travel and health* is the result of an extensive revision. After many years of annual updates covering technical details, the book has now been redesigned to better meet the needs of contemporary travellers. It is addressed primarily to medical and public health professionals who provide health advice to travellers, but it is also intended to provide guidance to travel agents and organizers, airlines and shipping companies. As far as possible, the information is presented in a form readily accessible to interested travellers and non-medical readers. For medical professionals, to whom other sources of additional details are available, essential information is given as concisely as possible.

In this new edition, there are some significant changes both in the scope of information provided and in its presentation. The book is intended to give guidance on the full range of significant health issues associated with travel. The roles of the medical profession, the travel industry and travellers themselves in avoiding health problems are recognized. The recommendations address the health risks associated with different types of travel and travellers. Business travel has increased dramatically, with frequent travellers now forming a substantial proportion of the total. Large numbers of travellers move far beyond the customary leisure and business centres, both for professional purposes and for pleasure, and there are now more elderly travellers, some of whom have pre-existing health problems. The risks and precautions specifically concerning infants and young children who travel also require special attention.

In this edition, air travel and its associated health risks receive greater emphasis, reflecting the enormous recent expansion in travel by air, particularly in long-haul flights. More information is given on environmental factors that may have adverse effects on travellers' health and well-being. The main infectious diseases that pose potential health threats for travellers are described individually, with the corresponding preventive measures. The worldwide distribution of the major infectious diseases is shown in maps, and—where possible—extensive text has been replaced by lists and tables. A separate chapter is devoted to information on the vaccine-preventable diseases and the corresponding vaccines, as well as guidance on the selection of vaccines for individual travellers. Sources of additional information are included with each chapter.

These and other changes in *International travel and health* have been made to facilitate its use and to focus on key information and clarity of presentation. An Internet version (http://www.who.int/ith) will allow updating during the year and provide easy links to other information, such as news of current disease outbreaks of international importance.

CHAPTER 1

Health risks and precautions: general considerations

People in their home environment live in a state of equilibrium with the locally occurring strains of microorganisms and with the altitude and climatic conditions of the region. However, this is an unstable equilibrium that can be upset even in the home environment by factors such as the arrival of an unfamiliar microorganism, seasonal changes in climate and unusually stressful situations. The many physical and environmental changes encountered during international travel may upset this equilibrium to an even greater extent: sudden exposure to significant changes in altitude, humidity, microbial flora and temperature, exacerbated by stress and fatigue, may result in ill-health and an inability to achieve the purpose of the journey. The risks associated with international travel are influenced by characteristics of the traveller (including age, sex and health status) and by characteristics of the travel (including destination, purpose and duration).

Forward planning, appropriate preventive measures and careful precautions can substantially reduce the risks of adverse health consequences. Although the medical profession and the travel industry can provide a great deal of help and advice, it is the traveller's responsibility to ask for information, to understand the risks involved, and to take the necessary precautions for the journey.

Travel-related risks

Key factors in determining the risks to which travellers may be exposed are:

— destination
— duration of visit
— purpose of visit
— standards of accommodation and food hygiene
— behaviour of the traveller.

Destinations where accommodation, hygiene and sanitation, medical care and water quality are of a high standard pose relatively few serious risks for the health of travellers, unless there is pre-existing illness. This applies to business travellers and tourists visiting most major cities and tourist centres and staying in good-quality accommodation. In contrast, destinations where accommodation is of poor quality, hygiene and sanitation are inadequate, medical services do not exist, and clean water is unavailable may pose serious risks for the health of travellers. This applies, for example, to personnel from emergency relief and development agencies or tourists who venture into remote areas. In these settings, stringent precautions must be taken to avoid illness.

The duration of the visit and the behaviour and lifestyle of the traveller are important in determining the likelihood of exposure to many infectious agents and will influence decisions on the need for certain vaccinations or antimalarial medication. The duration of the visit may also determine whether the traveller may be subjected to marked changes in temperature and humidity during the visit, or to prolonged exposure to atmospheric pollution.

The purpose of the visit is critical in relation to the associated health risks. A business trip to a city, where the visit is spent in a hotel and/or conference centre of high standard, or a tourist trip to a well-organized resort, involves fewer risks than a visit to remote rural areas, whether for work or pleasure. However, behaviour also plays an important role; for example, going outdoors in the evenings in a malaria-endemic area without taking precautions may result in the traveller becoming infected with malaria. Exposure to insects, rodents or other animals, infectious agents and contaminated food and water, combined with the absence of appropriate medical facilities, makes travel in many remote regions particularly hazardous.

Medical consultation before travel

Travellers intending to visit a destination in a developing country should consult a travel medicine clinic or medical practitioner before the journey. This consultation should preferably take place 4–6 weeks before the journey, particularly if vaccination(s) may be required. However, last-minute travellers can also benefit from a medical consultation, even as late as the day before travel. This consultation will determine the need for any vaccinations and/or antimalarial medication, as well as any other medical items that the traveller may require. A basic medical kit will be prescribed or provided, supplemented as appropriate to meet individual needs.

A dental check-up is advisable before travel to developing countries or prolonged travel to remote areas. This is particularly important for people with chronic or recurrent dental problems.

Assessment of health risks associated with travel

Medical advisers base their recommendations, including those for vaccinations and other medication, on an assessment of risk for the individual traveller, which takes into account the likelihood of catching a disease and how serious this might be for the traveller concerned. Key elements of this risk assessment are the destination, duration and purpose of the visit, as well as the conditions of accommodation and the health status of the traveller.

For each disease being considered, an assessment is also made of:

— availability of prophylaxis, possible side-effects and suitability for the traveller concerned;
— any associated public health risks (e.g. the risk of infecting others).

Collecting the information required to make a risk assessment involves detailed questioning of the traveller. A checklist or protocol is useful to ensure that all relevant information is obtained and recorded. The traveller should be provided with a personal record of the vaccinations given (patient-retained record) as vaccinations are often administered at different centres. A model checklist, reproducible for individual travellers, is provided on page 10.

Medical kit and toilet items

Sufficient medical supplies should be carried to meet all foreseeable needs for the duration of the trip.

A medical kit should be carried for all destinations where there may be significant health risks, particularly those in developing countries, and/or where the local availability of specific medications is not certain. This kit will include basic medicines to treat common ailments, first-aid articles, and any special medical items that may be needed by the individual traveller.

Certain categories of prescription medicine should be carried together with a medical attestation, signed by a physician, certifying that the traveller requires the medication for personal use. Some countries require not only a physician but also the national health administration to sign this certificate.

All medicines should be carried in the hand luggage to minimize any risk of loss during the journey. A duplicate supply carried in the checked luggage is a safety precaution in case of loss or theft.

Toilet items should also be carried in sufficient quantity for the entire visit unless their availability at the travel destination is assured. These will include items for dental care, eye care including contact lenses, skin care and personal hygiene.

Contents of a basic medical kit

First-aid items:

— adhesive tape
— antiseptic wound cleanser
— bandages
— emollient eye drops
— insect repellent
— insect bite treatment
— nasal decongestant
— oral rehydration salts
— scissors and safety pins
— simple analgesic (e.g. paracetamol)
— sterile dressing
— clinical thermometer.

Additional items according to destination and individual needs:

— antidiarrhoeal medication
— antifungal powder
— antimalarial medication
— condoms
— medication for any pre-existing medical condition
— sedatives
— sterile syringes and needles
— water disinfectant
— other items to meet foreseeable needs, according to the destination and duration of the visit.

Travellers with pre-existing medical conditions and special needs

Health risks associated with travel are greater for certain groups of travellers, including infants and young children, pregnant women, the elderly, the disabled, and those who have pre-existing health problems. For all of these travellers, medical advice and special precautions are necessary. They should be well informed about the available medical services at the travel destination.

Age

Infants and young children have special needs with regard to vaccinations and antimalarial precautions (see Chapters 6 and 7). They are particularly sensitive to ultraviolet radiation and become dehydrated more easily than adults in the event of inadequate fluid intake or loss of fluid due to diarrhoea. A child can be overcome by dehydration within a few hours. Air travel may cause discomfort to infants due to changes in cabin air pressure and is contraindicated for infants less than 7 days old. Infants and young children are more sensitive to sudden changes in altitude. They are also more susceptible to many infectious diseases.

Advanced age is not necessarily a contraindication for travel if the general health status is good. Elderly people should seek medical advice before planning long-distance travel.

Pregnancy

Travel is not generally contraindicated during pregnancy until close to the expected date of delivery, provided that the pregnancy is uncomplicated and the woman's health is good. Airlines impose some travel restrictions in late pregnancy and the neonatal period (see Chapter 2).

There are some restrictions on vaccination during pregnancy: specific information is provided in Chapter 6.

Pregnant women risk serious complications if they contract malaria. Travel to malaria-endemic areas should be avoided during pregnancy if at all possible. Specific recommendations for the use of antimalarial drugs during pregnancy are given in Chapter 7.

Medication of any type should be taken during pregnancy only in accordance with medical advice.

Travel to high altitudes (see also Chapter 3) or to remote areas is not advisable during pregnancy.

Disability

Physical disability is not usually a contraindication for travel if the general health status is good. Airlines have regulations on the conditions for travel for disabled passengers who need to be accompanied (see Chapter 2). Information should be obtained from the airline in advance.

Pre-existing illness

People suffering from chronic illnesses should seek medical advice before planning a journey. Conditions that increase health risks during travel include:

— cardiovascular disorders
— chronic hepatitis
— chronic inflammatory bowel diseases
— chronic renal disease requiring dialysis
— chronic respiratory diseases
— diabetes mellitus
— epilepsy
— immunosuppression due to medication or to HIV infection
— previous thromboembolic disease
— severe anaemia
— severe mental disorders
— any chronic condition requiring frequent medical intervention.

Any traveller with a chronic illness should carry all necessary medication for the journey and for the entire duration of the trip in their hand luggage. The name and contact details of their physician should be carried on their person with other travel documents, together with information about the medical condition and treatment, and details of medication (generic drug names included) and prescribed doses. A physician's letter certifying the necessity for any drugs or other medical items (e.g. syringes) carried by the traveller that may be questioned by customs officials should also be carried.

Insurance for travellers

International travellers should be aware that medical care abroad is often available only at private medical facilities and may be costly. In places where good-quality medical care is not readily available, travellers may need to be repatriated in case of accident or illness. If death occurs abroad, repatriation of the body can be extremely expensive and may be difficult to arrange. Travellers should be advised to (a) seek information about possible reciprocal health care agreements between the country of residence and the destination country, and (b) obtain special travellers' health insurance for destinations where health risks are significant and medical care is expensive or not readily available. This health insurance should include coverage for changes to the itinerary, emergency repatriation for health reasons, hospitalization, medical care in case of illness or accident and repatriation of the body in case of death.

Travel agents and tour operators usually provide information about travellers' health insurance. It should be noted that some countries now require proof of adequate health insurance as a condition for entry. Travellers should know the procedures to follow to obtain assistance and reimbursement. A copy of the insurance certificate and contact details should be carried with other travel documents in the hand luggage.

Role of travel industry professionals

Tour operators, travel agents, and airline and shipping companies each have an important responsibility to safeguard the health of travellers. It is in the interests of the travel industry that travellers have the fewest possible problems when travelling to, and visiting, foreign countries. Contact with travellers before the journey provides a unique opportunity to inform and advise them of the situation in each of the countries they are visiting. The travel agent or tour operator should provide the following health-related guidance to travellers:

- Advise the traveller to consult a travel medicine clinic as soon as possible after planning a trip to any destination where significant health risks may be foreseen, particularly those in developing countries, preferably 4–6 weeks before departure.

- Advise last-minute travellers that a visit should be made to a travel medicine clinic, even up to the day before departure.

- Advise travellers if the destination presents any particular hazards to personal safety and security and suggest appropriate precautions.

- Encourage travellers to take out comprehensive travellers' health insurance and provide information on available policies.

- Inform travellers of the procedures for obtaining assistance and reimbursement, particularly if the insurance policy is arranged by the travel agent or company.

- Provide information on:
  - mandatory vaccination requirements for yellow fever;
  - the need for malaria precautions at the travel destination;
  - the existence of other important health hazards at the travel destination;
  - the presence or absence of good-quality medical facilities at the travel destination.

Responsibility of the traveller

Travellers can obtain a great deal of information and advice from medical and travel industry professionals to help prevent health problems while abroad. However, travellers must accept that they are responsible for their health and well-being while travelling and on their return. The following are the main responsibilities to be accepted by the traveller:

— the decision to travel
— recognition and acceptance of any risks involved
— seeking health advice in good time, preferably 4–6 weeks before travel
— compliance with recommended vaccinations and other prescribed medication and health measures
— careful planning before departure
— carrying a medical kit and understanding its use
— obtaining adequate insurance cover
— health precautions before, during, and after the journey
— responsibility for obtaining a physician's letter pertaining to any prescription medicines, syringes, etc. being carried
— responsibility for the health and well-being of accompanying children
— precautions to avoid transmitting any infectious disease to others during and after travel
— careful reporting of any illness on return, including information about all recent travel
— respect for the host country and its population.

A model checklist for use by travellers, indicating steps to be taken before the journey, is provided on page 10.

Medical examination after travel

Travellers should be advised to have a medical examination on their return if they:

— suffer from a chronic disease, such as cardiovascular disease, diabetes mellitus, chronic respiratory disease;
— experience illness in the weeks following their return home, particularly if fever, persistent diarrhoea, vomiting, jaundice, urinary disorders, skin disease or genital infection occurs;
— consider that they have been exposed to a serious infectious disease while travelling;

— have spent more than 3 months in a developing country.

Travellers should provide medical personnel with information on recent travel, including destination, and purpose and duration of visit. Frequent travellers should give details of **all** journeys that have taken place in the preceding weeks and months.

Note. **Fever after returning from a malaria-endemic area is a medical emergency and travellers should seek medical attention immediately.**

Further reading

Dupont HL, Steffen R, eds. *Textbook of travel medicine and health*. London, BC Decker, 1997.

Zuckerman JN, ed. *Principles and practice of travel medicine*. Chichester, John Wiley & Sons, 2001.

Checklist for the traveller

Obtain information on local conditions

Depending on destination

- Risks related to the area (urban or rural)
- Type of accommodation (hotel, camping)
- Length of stay
- Altitude
- Security problems (e.g. conflict)
- Availability of medical facilities

Prevention

Vaccination. Contact the nearest travel medicine centre or a physician as early as possible, preferably 4–6 weeks before departure.

Malaria. Request appropriate preventive treatment and emergency reserves, and plan for bednet and insect repellent.

Food hygiene. Eat only thoroughly cooked food and drink only well-sealed bottled or packaged cold drinks. Boil drinking-water if safety is doubtful. If boiling is not possible, a certified well-maintained filter and/or disinfectant agent can be used.

Specific local diseases. Please consult the appropriate sections of this volume.

Accidents related to

- traffic (obtain a card showing blood group before departure)
- animals (beware of snakes and rabid dogs)
- allergies (use a medical alert bracelet)
- sun (pack sunglasses and sunscreen)

Get the following check-ups

- medical — obtain prescriptions for medication according to length of stay, and obtain advice from your physician on assembling a suitable medical kit
- dental
- ophthalmological — pack spare spectacles
- other according to specific conditions (e.g. pregnancy, diabetes)

Subscribe to a medical insurance with appropriate cover abroad, i.e. accident, sickness, medical repatriation.

Predeparture medical questionnaire

Surname: _____ First name: _____

Date of birth: _____ Country of origin: _____

Purpose of travel: ☐ Private ☐ Professional

Special activities: ☐ Accommodation: e.g. camping, bivouac

☐ Sports: e.g. diving, hunting, high-altitude trekking

Date of departure and length of stay : _____

Places to be visited

Country	Town	Rural area		Dates	
		Yes	No	From	to
		Yes	No	From	to
		Yes	No	From	to
		Yes	No	From	to
		Yes	No	From	to

Medical history: _____

Vaccination record: _____

Current state of health: _____

Chronic illnesses: _____

Recent or current medical treatment: _____

History of jaundice or hepatitis: _____

Allergies (e.g. eggs, antibiotics, sulfonamides): _____

For women: ☐ Current pregnancy

☐ Pregnancy likely within 3 months

☐ Currently breastfeeding

History of anxiety or depression: _____

☐ If yes, treatment prescribed (specify)

Neurological disorders (e.g. epilepsy, multiple sclerosis, etc.): _____

Cardiovascular disorders (e.g. thrombosis, use of pacemaker): _____

CHAPTER 2

Travel by air: health considerations

The volume of air traffic has risen steeply in recent years. The number of long-distance flights has increased greatly, and the distance that planes can fly non-stop, and therefore the duration of flights, also continues to rise. The passenger capacity of long-distance aircraft is increasing, so that larger numbers of people travel aboard a single aircraft. Frequent travellers now form a substantial proportion of the travelling public. According to the International Civil Aviation Organization, the annual number of flight passengers exceeded 1562 million in 1999 and 1647 million in 2000.

Air travel, particularly long-distance travel, exposes passengers to a number of factors that may adversely affect their health and well-being. Passengers with pre-existing health problems may find that they are more susceptible to these factors. Health risks associated with air travel can be minimized if the traveller plans carefully and takes some simple precautions before, during, and after the flight. An explanation of the various factors that may affect the health and well-being of air travellers follows.

Cabin air pressure

Although aircraft cabins are pressurized, cabin air pressure at cruising altitude is lower than air pressure at sea level. At a typical cruising altitude of 11 000 metres (37 000 feet), air pressure in the cabin is equivalent to that at an altitude of 1500–2500 metres (5000–8000 feet) above sea level. As a consequence, the available oxygen is reduced and gases within the body expand. The effects of reduced cabin air pressure are usually well tolerated by healthy passengers.

Oxygen and hypoxia

During all stages of flight, cabin air contains ample oxygen for healthy passengers. However, because cabin air pressure is relatively low, the oxygen saturation of the blood is slightly reduced, leading to mild hypoxia (i.e. reduced supply of oxygen to the tissues). Passengers with cardiovascular or respiratory disease, or certain disorders of the blood such as anaemia, may not tolerate hypoxia well. Moreover, the effect of alcohol on the brain is increased by hypoxia.

Gas expansion

Air expands in all air-filled body cavities as a result of the reduced cabin air pressure. Abdominal gas expansion may cause moderate discomfort, which may be exacerbated by consumption of carbonated beverages and certain vegetables. As the aircraft ascends, air escapes from the middle ear and the sinuses, usually without causing problems. As the aircraft descends, air must be allowed to flow back into the middle ear and sinuses in order to equalize pressure differences ("clearing the ears"). Most discomfort can be alleviated by swallowing, chewing, or yawning; if the problem persists, forceful expiration against a closed nose and mouth will usually help. For infants, feeding or giving a pacifier to stimulate swallowing may reduce the symptoms.

People with ear, nose, and sinus infections should avoid flying because pain and injury may result from the inability to equalize pressure differences. If travel cannot be avoided and problems arise during flight, decongestant nasal drops may be helpful.

Individuals who have recently undergone certain types of surgery should not fly for a period of time because of possible damage resulting from gas expansion (see page 22).

Cabin humidity

The relative humidity in aircraft cabins is low, usually less than 20%. Low humidity may cause discomfort of the eyes, mouth, and nose but presents little risk to health. Discomfort can be alleviated by maintaining good fluid intake before and during the flight, using a skin-moisturizing lotion, using a saline nasal spray to moisturize the nasal passages, and wearing spectacles rather than contact lenses.

Dehydration

Dehydration may develop during long flights unless adequate fluid intake is maintained. Fluid intake should consist of non-alcoholic beverages (water and fruit juices) both before and throughout the flight. As alcohol contributes to dehydration, consumption of alcohol should be restricted, and preferably avoided, before and during the flight.

Ozone and cosmic radiation

The concentration of ozone (triatomic oxygen, O_3) and the intensity of cosmic radiation both increase with altitude. Ozone is easily converted to oxygen by heat and various catalytic processes. In modern jet aircraft, almost all ozone in the ambient air is converted to oxygen in the compressors that provide pressurized air for the cabin. During descent, when engine power is low, a build-up of ozone is prevented by catalytic converters. At usual cruising altitudes, the concentration of ozone in the cabin air is negligible.

Cosmic radiation is the sum of solar and galactic radiation. At aviation altitudes, the cosmic ray field consists of low-ionizing radiation and neutrons. The atmosphere and the earth's magnetic field are natural shields. Because of the orientation of the magnetic field and the "flattening" of the atmosphere over the North and South Poles, cosmic radiation levels are significantly higher at polar than at equatorial latitudes. The intensity of cosmic radiation increases with altitude and is estimated to double about every 1500 metres (5000 feet). At usual cruising altitudes above 60°N (Canada, Scandinavia, etc.), an average radiation dose of about 0.3 mSv per 100 hours can be expected. For comparison, the natural background radiation from soil, water and building materials is about 2 mSv per year in most countries. The International Commission on Radiological Protection has set 1 mSv per year as a basic safety standard for the protection of the health of the general public against the dangers arising from additional ionizing radiation.

Motion sickness

Except in the case of severe turbulence, travellers by air rarely suffer from motion sickness. Travellers susceptible to motion sickness should request a seat over the wing and/or a window seat and keep the motion sickness bag provided readily accessible at all times. If necessary, medication may be taken to prevent motion sickness.

Immobility and circulatory problems

Prolonged immobility, particularly when the individual is seated, leads to pooling of blood in the legs, which in turn causes swelling, stiffness, and discomfort.

Circulatory stasis is a predisposing factor for the development of venous thrombosis (blood clots). In the case of air travel, it is possible, but not scientifically proven, that other factors in the flight environment also contribute.

Most venous thrombi do not cause any symptoms and are reabsorbed without any consequences. Occasionally, if a thrombus detaches from the lining of the vein and travels in the bloodstream to the lungs (pulmonary embolism), deep-vein thrombosis may have serious consequences including chest pain, shortness of breath, and even sudden death. This may occur many hours or even days after the formation of the thrombus.

The risk of developing deep-vein thrombosis is very small unless additional pre-existing risk factors for thromboembolism are present. These include:

— previous history of venous thrombosis
— age over 40 years (risk increases with age)
— use of estrogen therapy (oral contraceptives or hormone replacement therapy)
— pregnancy
— recent surgery or trauma, particularly abdominal or lower limb surgery
— cancer
— genetic blood-clotting abnormalities
— chronic venous insufficiency (varicose veins)
— congestive heart failure
— obesity.

It is advisable for people with one or more of these risk factors to seek medical advice before travelling.

Precautions

The negative effects of prolonged immobility can be reduced by doing simple exercises at frequent intervals during the flight. Many airlines provide helpful advice on in-flight exercises that stimulate the circulation, reduce discomfort, fatigue and stiffness, and lower the risk of developing venous thrombosis. Wearing graduated-compression stockings specially designed for air travel may be helpful. Hand luggage should not be placed where it may restrict movement of the legs and feet. Clothing should be loose and comfortable.

Based on evidence from its post-surgical use for prevention of thrombosis, aspirin is often advised for travellers taking long-distance flights. However, there is a need for research to determine whether aspirin has any protective effect for air travellers. Aspirin should not be used by travellers with medical contraindications, such as bleeding disorders or gastric ulcer, in view of the risk of adverse side-effects. Injection of low-molecular-weight heparin products may be prescribed for some high-risk travellers.

After arrival, the traveller can reduce the effects of the journey by gentle exercise to stimulate the circulation.

Jet lag

Jet lag refers to the disruption of sleep patterns and other circadian biorhythms (the body's internal clock) caused by crossing many time zones in a short period of time, e.g. when flying east–west or west–east. The adverse effects of jet lag are compounded by dehydration, fatigue and stress, and may lead to indigestion, general malaise, insomnia, and reduced physical and mental performance.

There are useful strategies for reducing the effects of jet lag (see below). Travellers who take medication according to a strict timetable (e.g. insulin, oral contraceptives) should seek medical advice.

General measures to reduce the effects of jet lag

- Be well rested before departure and have as much rest as possible during the flight, including short naps.
- Drink plenty of water and/or juices before and throughout the flight.
- Eat light meals and limit consumption of alcohol before and during the flight.
- Adjust to the destination time zone as quickly as possible (meal times, sleep time), preferably beginning during the flight.
- After arrival, ensure exposure to natural daylight.
- Short-acting sleeping pills may be helpful in assisting the adjustment of sleeping patterns after arrival; they should be used only in accordance with medical advice.[1]

Psychological aspects

Despite being an increasingly common mode of transport, travel by air is not a natural activity for human beings. Air travel is frequently accompanied by psychological difficulties. The main problems encountered are stress and fear of flying. These may occur together or separately at different times before and during the period of travel.

---

[1] Melatonin, at present available in very few countries (sold, but not approved by the Food and Drug Administration, in the USA) is used by some travellers to resynchronize the body's internal clock.

Flight phobia (fear of flying)

A considerable proportion of the general population in industrialized countries experiences some degree of fear of flying. This may have significant adverse effects on personal and professional life.

Flight phobia is often associated with the presence of other phobias, such as claustrophobia and agoraphobia. In addition, anxiety levels may be heightened by the presence of other stress-related factors, personality disorders or an underlying psychiatric disorder. Treatment is based on identification of the cause, and desensitization is the most commonly used intervention.

Travellers who experience fear of flying but are obliged to travel by air should seek medical advice before the journey. The use of tranquillizers or beta-blocking agents may be useful in some cases. Travellers taking tranquillizers should not consume alcohol. The dose of tranquillizer should not prevent arousal of the passenger in case of an emergency.

For longer-term treatment, travellers should be advised to seek specialized treatment to reduce the impact of psychological difficulties associated with air travel. Several airlines offer desensitization training courses to reduce or cure fear of flying.

Air rage

"Air rage" has been only relatively recently recognized as a form of disruptive behaviour associated with air travel. It appears to be linked to high levels of general stress but not specifically to flight phobia, and is frequently preceded by excessive consumption of alcohol.

Travellers with special needs

Individual airlines have different policies for the carriage of passengers with medical problems or those with special needs. Examples of commonly used guidelines are as follows.

Infants

Air travel is not recommended for infants less than 7 days old. For premature babies, medical advice should be sought in each case.

Changes in cabin air pressure may cause distress to infants, which can be alleviated by feeding or giving a pacifier to stimulate swallowing.

Infants are more susceptible to dehydration than older children and adults. Adequate fluid intake should be maintained before and during the flight. Extra fluid (water or diluted juice) should be provided periodically during long flights.

Pregnant women

Commercial flights are normally safe for mother and fetus. However, air travel is not recommended in the last month of pregnancy or until 7 days after delivery (see also page 22). Most airlines restrict acceptance of pregnant women. The common guidelines for uncomplicated pregnancy are:

— for single pregnancies, long-distance flying until the 36th week
— for multiple pregnancies, long-distance flying until the 32nd week.

A letter from a doctor or midwife confirming good health, normal pregnancy, and expected date of delivery should be carried after the 28th week of pregnancy. Medical clearance is required by some airlines for pregnant women if delivery is expected less than 4 weeks after the departure date or if any complications in delivery may be expected.

Pre-existing illness

People with diseases such as cancer, cardiovascular disorders, chronic respiratory disease, epilepsy, severe anaemia or unstable diabetes mellitus, and those who are taking immunosuppressive medication, are on renal dialysis, or whose fitness to travel is in doubt for any other reason should consult their doctor before deciding to travel by air. Medical clearance should be sought from the airline in case of doubt.

All medication for use during the journey and at the destination should be kept in the hand luggage and readily accessible at all times.

Flying is generally safe for passengers with pacemakers. Unipolar-lead pacing systems may be susceptible to electronic interference during flight and guidance on the effect of airport security screening devices should be obtained. Bipolar-lead pacing systems are not affected. However, hand-held security devices may interfere with implanted automatic defibrillators and travellers with these may find it useful to carry a physician's letter specifying this hazard.

Smokers

Smoking is banned on aircraft, except by a very few airlines. Smokers who regularly smoke heavily may experience stress and discomfort, particularly during long flights. Heavy smokers may benefit from medical advice before undertaking long-distance air travel. Nicotine-replacement patches or chewing-gum containing nicotine may be helpful and the use of a mild tranquillizer may be considered.

Travellers with disabilities

A physical disability is not usually a contraindication for travel. Passengers who are unable to look after their own needs during the flight (including use of the toilet and transfer from wheelchair to seat and vice versa) will need to be accompanied by a competent escort. Travellers confined to wheelchairs should be advised not to dehydrate themselves deliberately before travel (as a means of avoiding use of toilets during flights).

Airlines have regulations on conditions of travel for passengers with disabilities. Disabled passengers should contact the airline in advance for guidance.

Transmission of infectious diseases

Travellers should be reassured that there is very little risk of any infectious disease being transmitted on board the aircraft.

The quality of aircraft cabin air is carefully controlled. Exchange with outside air and filtration of recirculated cabin air provide a total change of air 20–30 times per hour. This level of ventilation is much greater than that in any building and ensures that contaminant levels are kept low. Modern aircraft recirculate up to 50% of cabin air. The recirculated air is passed through HEPA (high-efficiency particulate air) filters, which trap particulate material, bacteria, fungi and most viruses. Consequently, recirculated cabin air is very clean.

Transmission of airborne infectious agents between passengers is unlikely but may occasionally occur with those in close proximity to the source of infection. Influenza can be transmitted between passengers seated near each other. More widespread transmission of influenza may occur on board if the aircraft waits on the ground for an extended period with the ventilation system switched off. In a few instances, the tubercle bacillus (the organism that causes tuberculosis) has been transmitted to passengers seated close to a traveller suffering from tuberculosis. Most people do not develop any clinical disease as a result of infection by the tubercle bacillus, and in the case of the few infections transmitted on board the aircraft, none of the infected passengers developed the disease.

To avoid any risk of infecting others or transmitting disease from one country to another, as well as for personal health reasons, people with contagious diseases should not travel by air.

Aircraft disinsection

Many countries require disinsection (treatment for the removal of insects) of aircraft arriving from countries where vector-borne diseases such as malaria and yellow fever occur. This is to prevent the introduction of infection by insects inadvertently carried on board. Passengers may be infected by insects on board the aircraft and there have been a number of outbreaks of malaria in the vicinity of airports in countries where malaria is not present, owing to the escape of transported mosquitoes. Some countries, e.g. Australia and New Zealand, routinely carry out disinsection to prevent inadvertent introduction of species that may harm their agriculture.

Disinsection is a public health measure that is mandated by the International Health Regulations (see Annex 2, page 179). It involves treatment of the interior of the aircraft by the application of insecticides. The different procedures currently in use are as follows:

— treatment of the interior of the aircraft by application of a quick-acting pyrethroid insecticide spray, with the passengers on board, immediately before take-off;
— treatment of the interior of the aircraft on the ground before passengers come on board, using a residual insecticide aerosol containing permethrin, plus additional in-flight treatment with a quick-acting insecticide spray shortly before landing;
— regular application of a residual insecticide to all internal surfaces of the aircraft, except those in food-preparation areas.

Travellers are sometimes concerned about their exposure to insecticide sprays while travelling by air. There is anecdotal evidence of people feeling unwell in different ways after disinsection-spraying of aircraft. However, there is no evidence of a causal relationship between exposure to pyrethroids or other components of the sprays and the development of symptoms, provided that the recommended methods and products are used correctly for disinsection.

Medical assistance on board

Most airlines operating international flights have a policy for dealing with medical incidents on board and cabin crew are trained accordingly.

Large passenger aircraft usually carry the following emergency equipment and supplies:

— one or more first-aid kits, to be used by the crew;
— a medical kit, to be used by a medical doctor or other qualified persons to treat in-flight medical emergencies;
— an automated external defibrillator, to be used by the crew in case of cardiac emergencies.

In addition, some airlines are now equipped with medical diagnostic devices for transmitting clinical signs via the on-board telephone system to a medical expert at a ground-based response centre (telemedicine).

Cabin crew are trained in the use of first-aid materials and in carrying out first-aid and resuscitation procedures. They are usually also trained to recognize a range of medical conditions that may cause emergencies on board and to act appropriately to manage these.

Medical restrictions by airlines

Airlines require medical clearance by the medical department/adviser of the airline if there is an indication that a passenger may be suffering from any disease or physical or mental condition that may:

— adversely affect the welfare and comfort of the other passengers and/or crew members;
— be considered a potential hazard to the safety of the aircraft;
— require medical attention and/or special equipment during the flight;
— be aggravated by the flight.

Airlines reserve the right to refuse to carry passengers with conditions that may be exacerbated or cause serious consequences during the flight.

Frequent travellers who are permanently or chronically impaired may obtain a frequent traveller's medical card from the airline's medical department. This card is accepted, under specified conditions, as proof of medical clearance and for identification of the holder's impairment.

If cabin crew suspect, before departure, that a passenger may be ill, the aircraft's captain will be informed and a decision taken as to whether the passenger is fit to travel, needs medical attention, or presents a danger to other passengers or the safety of the aircraft.

Contraindications for air travel

Travel by air is contraindicated in the following cases:

- infants less than 7 days old;
- women in the last 4 weeks of pregnancy (8 weeks for multiple pregnancies) and until 7 days after delivery;[1]
- people suffering from:
  - angina pectoris or chest pain at rest
  - any serious or acute contagious disease
  - decompression sickness after diving[2]
  - increased intracranial pressure due to haemorrhage, trauma or infection
  - infections of the sinuses or infections of the ear and nose, particularly if the eustachian tube is blocked
  - recent myocardial infarction and stroke (time period depending on severity and duration of travel)
  - recent surgery or injury where trapped air or gas may be present, especially abdominal trauma and gastrointestinal surgery, cranio-facial and ocular injuries, brain operations, and eye operations involving penetration of the eyeball
  - severe chronic respiratory disease, breathlessness at rest, or unresolved pneumothorax
  - sickle-cell disease
  - uncontrolled arterial hypertension of more than 200 mmHg (27 kPa) systolic pressure.

Further reading

Schroeder E, Taudorf U, eds. *Air travel and transportation of patients: a guide for physicians*, 2nd ed. Copenhagen, Danish Armed Forces Health Services, 1997.

McNeil EL. *Airborne care of the ill and injured*. New York, Springer Verlag, 1983.

Martin T, Rodenberg HD. *Aeromedical transportation: a clinical guide*. Aldershot, Avebury Aviation, Ashgate Publishing Ltd, 1996.

---

[1] Subject to medical approval, travel may be permitted from 24 hours after delivery in case of exceptional need, provided that bleeding has stopped and haemoglobin levels are satisfactory.

[2] Scuba-divers should not fly too soon after diving: no earlier than 24 hours after multi-day unlimited scuba-diving, or 12 hours after a maximum of 2 hours of scuba-diving.

CHAPTER 3
Environmental health risks

Travellers often experience abrupt and dramatic changes in environmental conditions, which may have detrimental effects on health and well-being. Travel may involve major changes in altitude, temperature and humidity, and exposure to unfamiliar species of animals and insects. The negative impact of sudden changes in the environment can be minimized by taking simple precautions.

Altitude

At high altitude, atmospheric pressure is reduced. The consequent reduction in oxygen pressure can lead to hypoxia (i.e. reduced supply of oxygen to the tissues).

At altitudes of 1500–3500 metres, exercise tolerance is reduced and ventilation is increased. At 3500–5500 metres, there is hypoxia and altitude sickness may occur. Rapid ascent may lead to acute hypoxia: the affected person becomes faint and may lose consciousness. Acute mountain sickness may occur after 1–6 hours at high altitudes. Headache is followed by anorexia, nausea and vomiting, and insomnia, fatigue, lassitude, and irritability. The outcome is fatal in some cases due to the development of pulmonary and cerebral oedema.

Travellers with pre-existing cardiovascular or pulmonary disease or anaemia are highly sensitive to changes in altitude, which can be dangerous and even life-threatening.

Precautions for travellers unaccustomed to high altitudes

- Avoid direct travel to high altitudes if possible. Break the journey for 2–3 nights at 2500–3000 metres to help prevent acute mountain sickness.
- If direct travel to a high altitude cannot be avoided, the traveller should avoid overexertion, large meals, and alcohol after arrival.
- Travellers making a rapid ascent to high altitude (>3000 metres) can consider taking prophylactic medication (acetazolamide).
- Travellers planning to climb or trek at high altitude will require a period of gradual adaptation.

- Travellers with pre-existing cardiovascular or pulmonary disease or anaemia should seek medical advice before deciding to travel to a high altitude.

Heat and humidity

Sudden changes in temperature and humidity may have adverse effects on health. Exposure to high temperature and humidity results in loss of water and electrolytes (salts) and may lead to heat exhaustion and heat stroke. In hot dry conditions, dehydration is particularly likely to develop unless care is taken to maintain adequate fluid intake. The addition of a little table salt to food or drink (unless this is contraindicated for the individual) can help to prevent heat exhaustion, particularly during the period of adaptation.

Consumption of salt-containing food and drink helps to replenish the electrolytes in case of heat exhaustion and after excessive sweating. Older travellers should take particular care to consume extra fluids in hot conditions, as the thirst reflex diminishes with age. Care should be taken to ensure that infants and young children drink enough liquid to avoid dehydration.

Irritation of the skin may be experienced in hot conditions (prickly heat). Fungal skin infections such as tinea pedis (athlete's foot) are often aggravated by heat and humidity. A daily shower, wearing loose cotton clothing and applying talcum powder to sensitive skin areas help to reduce the development or spread of these infections.

Exposure to hot, dry, dusty air may lead to irritation and infection of the eyes and respiratory tract.

Ultraviolet radiation from the sun

The ultraviolet (UV) radiation from the sun includes UVA (wavelength 315–400 nm) and UVB (280–315 nm) radiation, both of which are damaging to human skin and eyes. The intensity of UV radiation is indicated by the Global Solar UV Index, which is a measure of skin-damaging radiation. The Index describes the level of solar UV radiation at the Earth's surface and is often reported as the maximum 10–30-minute average for the day. The values of the Index range from zero upwards—the higher the Index value, the greater the potential for damage to the skin and eyes, and the less time it takes for harm to occur. The Index values are grouped into exposure categories, with values greater than 10 being "extreme". In general, the closer to the equator the higher the Index. UVB radiation is particularly intense in summer and in the 4-hour period around solar noon. UV radiation may penetrate clear water to a depth of 1 metre or more.

The adverse effects of ultraviolet radiation from the sun are the following:

- Exposure to UV radiation, particularly UVB, can produce severe debilitating sunburn and sunstroke, particularly in light-skinned people.
- Exposure of the eyes may result in acute keratitis ("snow blindness"), and long-term damage leads to the development of cataracts.
- Long-term adverse effects on the skin include:
  — the development of skin cancers (carcinomas and malignant melanoma), mainly due to UVB radiation;
  — accelerated ageing of the skin, mainly due to UVA radiation, which penetrates more deeply into the skin.
- Adverse reactions of the skin result from interaction with a wide range of medicinal drugs that may cause photosensitization and result in phototoxic or photoallergic dermatitis. A variety of different types of therapeutic drugs as well as oral contraceptives, some prophylactic antimalarial drugs and certain antimicrobials may cause adverse dermatological reactions on exposure to sunlight. Phototoxic contact reactions are caused by topical application of products, including perfumes, containing oil of bergamot or other citrus oils.
- Exposure may suppress the immune system, increase the risk of infectious disease, and limit the efficacy of vaccinations.

Precautions

- Avoid exposure to the sun in the middle of the day, when the UV intensity is greatest.
- Wear clothing that covers arms and legs (summer clothing is UV-protective and generally more effective than even good-quality sunscreen).
- Wear UV-protective sunglasses of wrap-around design and a wide-brimmed sun hat.
- Apply a broad-spectrum sunscreen of sun protection factor (SPF) 15+ liberally on areas of the body not protected by clothing and reapply frequently.
- Take particular care to ensure that children are well protected.
- Take precautions against excessive exposure on or in water.
- Check that medication being taken will not affect sensitivity to UV radiation.

- If adverse skin reactions have occurred previously, avoid any exposure to the sun and avoid any products that have previously caused the adverse reactions.

Foodborne and waterborne health risks

Many important infectious diseases (such as brucellosis, cholera, crypto-sporidiosis, giardiasis, hepatitis A and E, legionellosis, leptospirosis, listeriosis, schistosomiasis and typhoid fever) are transmitted by contaminated food and water. Information on these and other specific infectious diseases of interest for travellers is provided in Chapter 5.

For travellers, the main health problem associated with contaminated food and water is "travellers' diarrhoea", which can be caused by a wide range of infectious agents. Travellers' diarrhoea is the most common health problem encountered by travellers and may affect up to 80% of travellers to high-risk destinations. Even a brief episode of severe diarrhoea may spoil a holiday or ruin a business trip. Diarrhoea may be accompanied by nausea, vomiting, and fever. Travellers' diarrhoea is primarily the result of consumption of contaminated food, drink, or drinking-water. Contamination in such cases is due to the presence of disease-producing microorganisms. A wide range of different bacteria, viruses, and some parasitic and fungal infections may cause travellers' diarrhoea.

Illness is also caused by certain biological toxins found in seafood. The main diseases in this group are caused by poisoning from:

— paralytic shellfish
— neurotoxic shellfish
— amnesic shellfish
— ciguatera toxin
— scombroid fish
— puffer fish.

The toxins involved in these poisonings come from microorganisms consumed by or otherwise contaminating the fish.

Poisonous chemicals may also contaminate food and drink. However, the ill-effects are generally the result of long-term exposure and do not represent a significant health risk for travellers. Sporadic misuse of chemicals also occurs, such as the use of textile dyes in foodstuffs, which may give an unusually bright colour to the contaminated food.

The safety of food, drink and drinking-water depends mainly on the standards of hygiene applied locally in their preparation and handling. In countries with low standards of hygiene and sanitation and poor infrastructure for controlling the safety of food, drink and drinking-water, there is a high risk of contracting travellers' diarrhoea. In such countries, travellers should take precautions with **all** food and drink, including that served in good-quality hotels and restaurants, to minimize any risk of contracting a foodborne or waterborne infection. While the risks are greater in poor countries, locations with poor hygiene may be present in any country.

Another potential source of waterborne infection is contaminated recreational water, particularly sewage-polluted seawater or fresh water in lakes and rivers, as well as water in swimming pools and spas where filtering and disinfection are inadequate or even non-existent. Bathing in contaminated water may result in ingestion of diarrhoea-producing microorganisms and other infectious agents.

It is particularly important that people in more vulnerable groups, i.e. infants and children, the elderly, pregnant women and people with impaired immune systems, take stringent precautions to avoid contaminated food and drink and unsafe recreational waters.

Travellers should:

— avoid consumption of potentially contaminated food or drink;
— avoid contact with potentially contaminated recreational waters;
— know how to treat diarrhoea;
— carry oral rehydration salts and water-disinfecting agents.

Precautions for avoiding unsafe food and drink

● Avoid cooked food that has been kept at room temperature for several hours.

● Eat only food that has been cooked thoroughly and is still hot.

● Avoid uncooked food, apart from fruit and vegetables that can be peeled or shelled, and avoid fruits with damaged skins.

● Avoid dishes containing raw or undercooked eggs.

● Avoid food bought from street vendors.

● Avoid ice cream from unreliable sources, including street vendors.

● In countries where poisonous biotoxins may be present in fish and shellfish, obtain advice locally.

● Boil unpasteurized (raw) milk before consumption.

- Boil drinking-water if its safety is doubtful; if boiling is not possible, a certified, well-maintained filter and/or a disinfectant agent can be used.

- Avoid ice unless it has been made from safe water.

- Avoid brushing the teeth with unsafe water.

- Bottled or packaged cold drinks are usually safe provided that they are sealed; hot beverages are usually safe.

Intestinal parasites: risks for travellers

Travellers, particularly those visiting tropical and subtropical countries, may be exposed to a number of intestinal parasitic helminth (worm) infections. The risk of acquiring intestinal parasites is associated with low standards of hygiene and sanitation, which permit contamination of soil, sand and foodstuffs with human or canine faeces. In general, the clinical effects are likely to become apparent some time after return from travel and the link with the travel destination may not be apparent, which in turn may delay the diagnosis or lead to misdiagnosis. The following are the main intestinal parasitic helminths to which travellers may be exposed.

■ **Hookworms**. Human and canine hookworms, particularly *Necator* and *Ancylostoma* species, may be a risk for travellers, notably in places where beaches are polluted by human or canine faeces. Humans become infected by larval forms of the parasite which penetrate the skin. *A. caninum* produces a characteristic skin lesion, cutaneous larval migrans, which is readily treated by anthelminthics such as albendazole.

■ **Tapeworms**. The tapeworm *Taenia saginata* is acquired by consumption of raw or undercooked beef from cattle that harbour the larval form of the parasite. *T. solium* is similarly acquired from raw or undercooked pork. These tapeworm infections result from access of cattle and pigs to human faeces, from which they ingest tapeworm eggs. *T. solium* infection in humans may also result from ingestion of *T. solium* eggs in food contaminated by faeces; this is particularly dangerous, since the larval forms of the parasite cause cysticercosis, which may produce serious disease. The tapeworm *Echinococcus granulosus* causes cystic hydatid disease due to infection by the larval form of the parasite; the adult tapeworms infect dogs, which excrete eggs in the faeces. Human infection is acquired by ingestion of eggs following close contact with infected dogs or consumption of food or water contaminated by their faeces.

■ **Roundworms**. The intestinal roundworm (nematode) parasites *Ascaris* and *Trichuris* are transmitted in soil. Soil containing eggs of these parasites may contaminate foods such as fruit and vegetables, leading to infection if the food is consumed without thorough washing; infection may also be transmitted by the hands following handling of soil-contaminated foods, for instance in street markets.

Precautions for avoiding unsafe recreational waters

- Seek information locally about the quality of recreational waters in the area.
- Avoid beaches obviously polluted by sewage.
- Avoid bathing in sewage-contaminated water.
- Avoid swallowing any sewage-contaminated water.

Treatment of diarrhoea

- Most diarrhoeal attacks are self-limiting, with recovery in a few days. It is important, especially for children, to avoid becoming dehydrated.
- As soon as diarrhoea starts, more fluids should be taken, such as bottled, boiled or treated water, or weak tea. If diarrhoea continues for more than one day, oral rehydration salt (ORS) solution should be taken and normal food consumption should continue.

Amounts of ORS solution to drink

Children under 2 years $^{1}/_{4}$–$^{1}/_{2}$ cup (50–100 ml) after each loose stool

Children 2–10 years $^{1}/_{2}$–1 cup (100–200 ml) after each loose stool

Older children and adults   Unlimited amount

If ORS solution is not available, a substitute containing 6 level teaspoons of sugar plus 1 level teaspoon of salt in 1 litre of safe drinking-water can be used, in the same amounts as for ORS. (A level teaspoon contains a volume of 5 ml.)

Medical help should be sought if diarrhoea lasts for more than 3 days and/or there are very frequent watery bowel movements, blood in the stools, repeated vomiting or fever.

When no medical help is available and there is blood in the stools, a course of ciprofloxacin may be taken by adults. For children and pregnant women, azithromycin is recommended. Prophylactic use of antimicrobials is not recommended. Antidiarrhoeal medicines, e.g. loperamide, are not recommended for general use but may be used exceptionally, in addition to fluids and by adults only, for symptomatic relief. Antidiarrhoeal medicines should never be used to treat children.

If there are other symptoms, medical advice should be sought.

Recreational waters

The use of coastal waters and freshwater lakes and rivers for recreational purposes has a beneficial effect on health through exercise, and rest and relaxation. However, various hazards to health may also be associated with recreational waters. The main risks are the following:

- Drowning and injury (see Chapter 4).
- Physiological:
  — chilling, leading to coma and death;
  — thermal shock, leading to cramps and cardiac arrest;
  — acute exposure to heat and ultraviolet radiation in sunlight: heat exhaustion, sunburn, sunstroke;
  — cumulative exposure to sun (skin cancers, cataract).
- Infection:
  — ingestion or inhalation of, or contact with, pathogenic bacteria, fungi, parasites and viruses;
  — bites by mosquitoes and other insect vectors of infectious diseases.
- Poisoning and toxicoses:
  — ingestion or inhalation of, or contact with, chemically contaminated water, including oil slicks;
  — stings or bites of venomous animals;
  — ingestion or inhalation of, or contact with, blooms of toxigenic plankton.

Exposure to cold: immersion hypothermia

Cold, rather than simple drowning, is the main cause of death at sea. When the body temperature falls (hypothermia), there is confusion followed by loss of consciousness, so that the head goes under water leading to drowning. With a life jacket capable of keeping the head out of water, drowning is avoided, but death due directly to hypothermic cardiac arrest will soon follow. However, wearing warm clothing as well as a life jacket can greatly prolong survival in cold water. Children, particularly boys, have less fat than adults and chill very rapidly in cool or cold water.

Swimming is difficult in very cold water (around 0°C), and even good swimmers often drown suddenly if they attempt to swim even short distances in water at these temperatures without a life jacket. Life jackets or some other form of flotation aid should always be worn in small craft, particularly by children and young men, when the water is cold.

Alcohol, even in small amounts, can cause hypoglycaemia if consumed without food and after exercise. It causes confusion and disorientation and also, in cold surroundings, a rapid fall in body temperature. Unless sufficient food is eaten at the same time, small amounts of alcohol can be exceedingly dangerous on long-distance swims, as well as after rowing or other strenuous and prolonged water-sports exercise.

Those engaging in winter activities on water, such as skating and fishing, should be aware that whole-body immersion must be avoided. Accidental immersion in water at or close to freezing temperatures is dangerous because the median lethal immersion time (time to death) is less than 30 minutes for children and most adults.

Immediate treatment is much more important than any later action in reviving victims of immersion hypothermia. A hot bath (the temperature no higher than the immersed hand will tolerate) is the most effective method of achieving this. In case of drowning, cardiac arrest and cessation of breathing should be treated by tipping water out of the stomach and giving immediate external cardiac massage and artificial ventilation. Cardiac massage should not be applied unless the heart has stopped. People who have inhaled water should always be sent to hospital to check for pulmonary complications.

Infection

In coastal waters, infection may result from ingestion or inhalation of, or contact with, pathogenic microorganisms, which may be naturally present, carried by people or animals using the water, or present as a result of faecal contamination. The most common consequences among travellers are diarrhoeal disease, acute febrile respiratory disease and ear infections.

In fresh waters, leptospirosis may be spread by the urine of infected rodents, causing human infection through contact with broken skin or mucous membranes. In areas endemic for schistosomiasis, infection may be acquired by penetration of the skin by larvae during swimming or wading. (See also Chapter 5.)

In swimming pools and spas, infection may occur if treatment and disinfection of the water is inadequate. Diarrhoea, gastroenteritis and throat infections may result from contact with contaminated water. Appropriate use of chlorine and other disinfectants controls most viruses and bacteria in water. However, the parasites *Giardia* and *Cryptosporidium*, which are shed in large numbers by infected individuals, are highly resistant to routine disinfection procedures. They are inactivated by ozone or eliminated by filtration.

Contamination of spas and whirlpools may lead to infection by *Legionella* and *Pseudomonas aeruginosa*. Otitis externa and infections of the urinary tract, respiratory tract, wounds and cornea have also been linked to spas.

Direct person-to-person contact or physical contact with contaminated surfaces in the vicinity of pools and spas may spread the viruses that cause molluscum contagiosum and cutaneous papillomas (warts); fungal infections of the hair, fingernails and skin, notably tinea pedis (athlete's foot), are spread in a similar manner.

Precautions

- Adopt safe behaviour in all recreational waters (see Chapter 4).
- Avoid consumption of alcohol before any activities in or near recreational waters.
- Provide constant supervision of children in the vicinity of recreational waters.
- Avoid temperature extremes in spas, saunas, etc.; this is particularly important for users with pre-existing medical conditions, pregnant women and young children.
- Avoid excessive exposure to sunlight.
- Avoid contact with contaminated waters.
- Avoid swallowing any contaminated water.
- Obtain advice locally about the presence of potentially dangerous aquatic animals.
- Wear shoes when walking on shores, riverbanks and muddy terrain.

Animals and insects

Mammals

Animals tend to avoid contact with humans and most do not attack unless provoked. Some large carnivores, however, are aggressive and may attack. Animals suffering from rabies often become aggressive and may attack without provocation. Wild animals may become aggressive if there is territorial intrusion, particularly when the young are being protected. Animal bites may cause serious injury and may also result in transmission of disease.

Rabies is the most important infectious health hazard from animal bites. In many developing countries, rabies is transmitted mainly by dogs, but many other species of mammals can be infected by the rabies virus. After any animal bite, the wound should be thoroughly cleansed with disinfectant or with soap or detergent and water, and medical or veterinary advice should be sought about the possibility of rabies in the area. Where a significant risk of rabies exists, the patient should be treated with post-exposure rabies vaccination and immunoglobulin (see Chapter 5). A booster dose of tetanus toxoid is also recommended following an animal bite.

Travellers who may be at increased risk of exposure to rabies may be advised to have pre-exposure vaccination before departure (see Chapter 6). Pre-exposure rabies vaccination does not eliminate the need for treatment after the bite of a rabid animal, but it reduces the number of vaccine doses required in the post-exposure regimen.

Precautions
- Avoid direct contact with domestic animals in areas where rabies occurs, and with all wild and captive animals.
- Avoid behaviour that may startle, frighten or threaten an animal.
- Ensure that children do not approach, touch, or otherwise provoke any animal.
- Treat any animal bite immediately by washing with disinfectant or soap and seek medical advice.
- If a significant risk of exposure to rabies is foreseen, seek medical advice before travelling.

Travellers with accompanying animals should be aware that dogs (and, for some countries, cats) must be vaccinated against rabies in order to be allowed to cross international borders. A number of rabies-free countries have additional requirements. Before taking an animal abroad, the traveller should ascertain the regulatory requirements of the countries of destination and transit.

Snakes, scorpions and spiders
Travellers to tropical, subtropical and desert areas should be aware of the possible presence of venomous snakes, scorpions and spiders. Local advice should be sought about risks in the areas to be visited. Most venomous species are particularly active at night.

Venom from snake and spider bites and from scorpion stings have various effects in addition to tissue damage in the vicinity of the bite. Neurotoxins are present in the venom of both terrestrial and aquatic snakes, and also often in the venom of scorpions and spiders. Neurotoxins cause weakness and paralysis and other symptoms. Venom contacting the eyes causes severe damage and may result in blindness. Most snake venoms affect blood coagulation, which may result in haemorrhage and reduced blood pressure. Toxins in the hair of spiders such as tarantulas may cause intense irritation on contact with the skin.

Poisoning by a venomous snake, scorpion or spider is a medical emergency requiring immediate attention. The patient should be moved to the nearest medical facility as quickly as possible. First-aid measures call for immobilizing the entire affected limb with splints and firm, but not tight, bandaging to limit the spread of toxin in the body and the amount of local tissue damage. However, bandaging is not recommended if local swelling and tissue damage are present in the vicinity of the bite. Other traditional first-aid methods (incisions and suction, tourniquets and compression) are harmful and should not be used.

The decision to use antivenom should be taken only by qualified medical personnel, and it should be administered in a medical facility. Antivenom should be given only if its stated range of specificity includes the species responsible for the bite.

Precautions

- Obtain local advice about the possible presence of venomous snakes, scorpions and spiders in the area.
- Avoid walking barefoot or in open sandals in terrain where venomous snakes, scorpions or spiders may be present; wear boots or closed shoes and long trousers.
- Avoid placing hands or feet where snakes, spiders or scorpions may be hiding.
- Be particularly careful outdoors at night.
- Examine clothing and shoes before use for hidden snakes, scorpions or spiders.

Aquatic animals

Swimmers and divers may be bitten by certain aquatic animals, including conger and moray eels, stingrays, weever fish, scorpionfish, stonefish, piranhas, seals and sharks. They may be stung by venomous cnidaria—jellyfish, fire corals, sea anemones—and other invertebrate aquatic species including octopus. Severe and often fatal injury results from attack by crocodiles, which inhabit rivers and estuaries in many tropical countries, including the tropical north of Australia. Injuries from dangerous aquatic organisms occur as a result of:

— passing close to a venomous organism while bathing or wading;
— treading on a stingray, weever fish or sea urchin;
— handling venomous organisms during sea-shore exploration;
— invading the territory of large animals when swimming or at the water's edge;
— swimming in waters used as hunting grounds by large predators;
— interfering with, or provoking, dangerous aquatic organisms.

Precautions

● Obtain local advice on the possible presence of dangerous aquatic animals in the area.

● Adopt behaviour that will avoid provoking attack by predatory animals.

● Wear shoes when walking on the shore and at the water's edge.

● Avoid contact with jellyfish in water and dead jellyfish on the beach.

● Avoid walking, wading or swimming in crocodile-infested waters at all times of year.

● Seek medical advice after a sting or bite by a poisonous animal.

Treatment

In the case of envenomings by aquatic animals, treatment will depend on whether there is a wound or puncture or a localized skin reaction (e.g. rash). Punctures caused by spiny fish require immersion in hot water, extraction of the spines, careful cleaning of the wound and antibiotic therapy (and antivenom in the case of stonefish). If punctures were caused by an octopus or sea urchin the treatment is basically the same but without exposure to heat. In the case of rashes or linear lesions, contact with cnidaria should be suspected; the treatment is based on the use of 5% acetic acid, local decontamination and corticosteroids (antivenom for the box jellyfish *Chironex fleckeri*), with adequate follow-up for eventual sequelae.

Insects and other vectors of disease

Vectors play an essential role in the transmission of many infectious diseases. Many vectors are bloodsucking insects, which ingest the disease-producing microorganism during a blood meal from an infected host (human or animal) and later inject it into a new host at the time of another blood meal. Mosquitoes are important insect vectors of disease, and some diseases are transmitted by bloodsucking flies. In addition, ticks and certain aquatic snails are involved in the life cycle and transmission of disease. The principal vectors and the main diseases they transmit are shown in Table 3.1 at the end of this chapter. Information about the diseases and specific preventive measures are provided in Chapters 5, 6 and 7.

The geographical distribution of vector-borne diseases depends on the ecological requirements of the vector. Water plays a key role for most vectors. Thus, the transmission of many vector-borne diseases is seasonal since it depends on rainfall. Temperature is also a critical factor, limiting the distribution of vectors by altitude and latitude.

Exposure of travellers to vectors is influenced by the purpose of the visit. Business travellers on short visits (less than 2 weeks) to urban centres may be exposed to the vectors of dengue, which bite mostly during the day, but are otherwise at relatively low risk of exposure to vector-borne diseases.

Leisure travellers may be exposed to vectors in non-air-conditioned hotels, during early evenings outdoors, or during visits to sites outside the urban environment.

Adventure travellers seeking pristine ecosystems have a relatively high risk of exposure to disease vectors and personal protection is essential.

Backpackers and tourists on safari have a high risk of exposure to vectors and personal protection is required. Backpackers often spend longer and live in closer contact with local populations than other visitors. Exposure to vectors is one of several health risks in environments with low standards of hygiene and sanitation.

Protection against vectors

Travellers may protect themselves from mosquitoes and other vectors by the means outlined in the following paragraphs.

Insect repellents are substances applied to exposed skin or to clothing to prevent human/vector contact. The active ingredient in a repellent, usually diethyl-toluamide (DEET), repels but does not kill insects. Neck, wrists and ankles are target areas for application, and care must be taken to avoid contact with mucous membranes. Insect repellents should not be sprayed on the face or applied to the eyelids or lips. They should not be applied to sensitive, sunburned or damaged skin or deep skin folds. When the product is applied on the skin, the repellent effect may last from 15 minutes to 10 hours, depending on a number of factors including climate and humidity, the formulation of the product, and the vector species. Repeated application may therefore be necessary. When the product is applied to clothes, the repellent effect is longer. It is recommended that the use of repellents in the early evening should be combined with sleeping under a mosquito net. Repellents should be used in strict accordance with the manufacturers' instructions and the dosage must not be exceeded, especially for young children.

Mosquito coils are the best known example of insecticide vaporizer, usually with a synthetic pyrethroid as the active ingredient. One coil serves a normal bedroom through the night, unless the room is particularly draughty. A more sophisticated version, which requires electricity, is an insecticide mat that is placed on an electrically heated grid, causing the insecticide to evaporate.

Insecticide sprays are effective for an immediate knockdown and killing effect. They contain an insecticide and a propellant to create an aerosol in a room. Indoor sleeping areas should be sprayed before bedtime. There is little or no residual effect, however; treating a room with an insecticide spray will help to free it from insects, but the effect may be short-lived. Spraying combined with the use of a coil or vaporizer or of a mosquito net is recommended.

Protective clothing can be effective outdoors at times of the day when vectors are active. The thickness of the material is critical, and no skin should be left exposed unless treated with a repellent. Insect repellent applied to clothing is effective for longer than it may be on the skin. Extra protection is provided by treating clothing with permethrin or etofenprox, to prevent mosquitoes from biting through clothing. Label instructions should be followed to avoid damage to certain fabrics. Boots are useful to protect the feet in tick-infested areas, combined with a repellent.

Mosquito nets are the best solution for most travellers. Nets can be used either with or without insecticide impregnation. Impregnated nets are much more effective. Commercially available nets are impregnated with insecticides belonging to the group of synthetic pyrethroids. Mesh size and strength are crucial characteristics: the mesh size should be less than 1.5 mm. In some malarious countries, hotel rooms in endemic zones will have mosquito nets permanently installed. These should be checked for holes, and they can be temporarily re-impregnated using a synthetic pyrethroid spray. It is important to use the mosquito net correctly. The net should be tucked in under the mattress, ensuring first that it has no holes and that there are no mosquitoes inside. Nets for use with cots and small beds are available. Babies should be kept under insecticide-treated mosquito nets as much as possible between dusk and dawn.

Travellers camping in tents should use a combination of mosquito coils, repellents and screens. The mesh size of tent screens often exceeds 1.5 mm, so that special mosquito screens have to be deployed.

Screening of windows, doors and eaves is a solution for travellers who are staying in one location for some time, or for those on emergency and humanitarian aid missions.

Table 3.1 **Principal disease vectors and the diseases they transmit**[a]

Vectors	Main diseases transmitted
Aquatic snails	Schistosomiasis (bilharziasis)
Blackflies	River blindness (onchocerciasis)
Fleas	Plague (transmitted by fleas from rats to humans)
Mosquitoes	
Aedes	Dengue fever
	Rift Valley fever
	Yellow fever
Anopheles	Lymphatic filariasis
	Malaria
Culex	Japanese encephalitis
	Lymphatic filariasis
	West Nile fever
Sandflies	Leishmaniasis
	Sandfly fever (*Phlebotomus* fever)
Ticks	Crimean–Congo haemorrhagic fever
	Lyme disease
	Relapsing fever (borreliosis)
	Rickettsial diseases including spotted fevers and Q fever
	Tick-borne encephalitis
	Tularaemia
Triatomine bugs	Chagas disease (American trypanosomiasis)
Tsetse flies	Sleeping sickness (African trypanosomiasis)

[a] Based on extensive research, there is absolutely no evidence that HIV infection can be transmitted by insects.

Air-conditioning is a highly effective means of keeping mosquitoes and other insects out of a room. In air-conditioned hotels, other precautions are not necessary indoors.

Contact with fresh water (lakes, slow-running streams) is to be avoided in areas where schistosomiasis is prevalent. For occupational contact (for example, irrigation consultants visiting an affected area), protective boots are recommended.

Further reading

WHO advice on sun protection: http://www.who.int/peh-uv/sunprotection.htm

Foodborne disease: a focus on health education. Geneva, WHO, 2000. (See annex for comprehensive information on 31 foodborne diseases caused by bacteria, viruses and parasites.)

WHO guide on safe food for travellers: http://www.who.int/fsf/brochure/trvl1.htm

WHO guidelines for safe recreational-water environments. http://www.who.int/water_sanitation_health/Recreational_water/eosdraft9814.htm (Vol. 1 – Coastal and freshwaters; Vol. 2 – Swimming pools, spas and similar recreational-water environments).

Bites and stings due to terrestrial and aquatic animals in Europe: http://www.who.int/wer/pdf/2001/wer7638.pdf

Vectors of disease, Part I: http://www.who.int/wer/pdf/2001/wer7625.pdf

Vectors of disease, Part II: http://www.who.int/wer/pdf/2001/wer7626.pdf

Rozendaal J. *Vector control: methods for use by individuals and communities.* Geneva, WHO, 1997.

CHAPTER 4

Accidents, injuries and violence

Travellers are more likely to be killed or injured in accidents or through violence than to be struck down by an exotic infectious disease. Traffic accidents are the most frequent cause of death among travellers. Traffic accidents and violence are significant risks in many countries, particularly developing countries, where skilled medical care may not be readily available. Accidents and injuries also occur in other settings, particularly in recreational waters in association with swimming, diving, sailing and other activities. Travellers can reduce the possibility of incurring these risks through awareness of the dangers and by taking the appropriate precautions.

Traffic accidents

It is estimated that more than 1 million people were killed in traffic accidents worldwide in 1998 and a further 10 million were injured.

In many developing countries traffic laws are limited or are inadequately enforced. Often the traffic mix is more complex than that in developed countries and involves two- and four-wheeled vehicles, animal-drawn vehicles and other conveyances, plus pedestrians, all sharing the same road space. The roads may be poorly constructed and maintained, road signs and lighting inadequate and driving habits poor. Travellers, both drivers and pedestrians, should be extremely attentive and careful on the roads.

There are a number of practical precautions that travellers can take to reduce the risk of being involved in, or becoming the victim of, a traffic accident.

Precautions

- Have full insurance cover for medical treatment of both illness and injuries sustained in accidents.
- Carry an international driving licence as well as your national driving licence.

- Obtain information on the regulations governing traffic and vehicle maintenance, and on the state of the roads, in the countries to be visited.

- Before renting a car check the state of the tyres, safety belts, spare wheels, lights, brakes, etc.

- Know the informal rules of the road; in some countries, for example, it is customary to sound the horn or flash the headlights before overtaking.

- Be particularly vigilant in a country where the traffic drives on the opposite side of the road to that used in your country of residence.

- Do not drive on unfamiliar and unlit roads.

- Do not use a moped, motorcycle or bicycle.

- Do not drive after drinking alcohol.

- Drive within the speed limit at all times.

- Always wear a safety belt where these are available.

- Beware of wandering animals.

Injuries and accidents in recreational waters

Recreational waters include coastal waters, freshwater lakes and rivers, swimming pools and spas. The hazards associated with recreational waters can be minimized by safe behaviour and simple precautions.

The most important health hazards in recreational waters are drowning and impact injuries, particularly head and spinal injuries. It is estimated that at least half a million deaths are caused by drowning every year. In addition, many more cases of "near-drowning" occur, often with life-long effects on health.

Drowning may occur when a person is caught in a tide or rip current, is trapped by rising tides, falls overboard from a boat, becomes caught in submerged obstacles, or falls asleep on an inflatable mattress and is carried out to sea. In swimming pools and spas, drowning or near-drowning and other injuries may occur close to outlets where suction is strong enough to catch body parts or hair so that the head is trapped under water. Drowning in swimming pools may be related to slip–trip–fall accidents leading to loss of consciousness on impact. If the water is not clear it may be difficult to see submerged swimmers or obstacles, increasing the chances of an accident in the water.

Children can drown in a very short time and in relatively small amounts of water. The factor that contributes most frequently to children drowning is lack of adult supervision. Children in or near water should be constantly supervised by adults.

Drowning is also a hazard for those wading and fishing. Falling in cold water, particularly when wearing heavy clothing, may result in drowning as swimming ability is hampered.

Impact injuries are usually the result of diving accidents, particularly diving into shallow water and/or hitting underwater obstructions. Water may appear to be deeper than it is. Impact of the head on a hard surface may cause head and/or spinal injuries. Spinal injuries may result in various degrees of paraplegia or quadriplegia. Head injuries may cause concussion and loss of memory and/or motor skills.

Drowning and impact injuries in adults are frequently associated with alcohol consumption, which impairs judgement and the ability to react effectively.

A detached retina, which can result in blindness or near-blindness, may be caused by jumping into water or jumping onto other people in the water.

Precautions

- Adopt safe behaviour in all recreational waters: use life jackets where appropriate, pay attention to tides and currents, and avoid outlets in spas and swimming pools.

- Ensure constant adult supervision of children in or near recreational waters, including small volumes of water.

- Avoid consumption of alcohol before any activity in or near water.

- Check the depth of the water carefully before diving, and avoid diving or jumping into murky water as submerged swimmers or objects may not be visible.

- Do not jump into water or jump onto others in the water.

Violence

Violence is a significant risk in many developing countries. Criminals often target tourists and business travellers, particularly in countries where crime levels are high. However, some sensible precautions may reduce this risk.

Precautions

- Be alert to muggings during the day as well as at night.
- Keep jewellery, cameras and other items of value out of sight and do not carry large sums of money on your person.
- Avoid isolated beaches and other remote areas.
- Avoid overcrowded trains, buses and minibus taxis.
- Use taxis from authorized ranks only.
- Avoid driving at night and never travel alone.
- Keep car doors locked and windows shut.
- Be particularly alert when waiting at traffic lights.
- Park in well-lit areas and do not pick up strangers.
- Employ the services of a local guide/interpreter or local driver when travelling to remote areas.
- Vehicle hijacking is a recognized risk in a number of countries. If stopped by armed robbers, make no attempt to resist and keep hands where the attackers can see them at all times.

Further reading

WHO information on violence and injury prevention: http://www.who.int/violence_injury_prevention/pubs.htm

CHAPTER 5

Infectious diseases of potential risk for travellers

Depending on the travel destination, travellers may be exposed to a number of infectious diseases; exposure depends on the presence of infectious agents in the area to be visited. The risk of becoming infected will vary according to the purpose of the trip and the itinerary within the area, the standards of accommodation, hygiene and sanitation, as well as the behaviour of the traveller. In some instances, disease can be prevented by vaccination, but there are some infectious diseases, including some of the most important and most dangerous, for which no vaccines exist.

General precautions can greatly reduce the risk of exposure to infectious agents and should always be taken for visits to any destination where there is a significant risk of exposure. These precautions should be taken regardless of whether any vaccinations or medication have been administered.

Modes of transmission and general precautions

The modes of transmission for different infectious diseases and the corresponding general precautions are outlined in the following paragraphs.

Foodborne and waterborne diseases

Food- and waterborne diseases are transmitted by consumption of contaminated food and drink. The risk of infection is reduced by taking hygienic precautions with all food, drink and drinking-water consumed when travelling and by avoiding direct contact with polluted recreational waters (see Chapter 3). Examples of diseases transmitted by food and water are hepatitis A, typhoid fever and cholera.

Vector-borne diseases

A number of particularly serious infections are transmitted by insects and other vectors such as ticks. The risk of infection can be reduced by taking precautions to avoid insect bites and contact with other vectors in places where infection is likely to be present (see Chapter 3). Examples of vector-borne diseases are malaria, yellow fever, dengue and tick-borne encephalitis.

Zoonoses (diseases transmitted from animals)

Zoonoses include many infections that can be transmitted to humans through animal bites or contact with contaminated body fluids or faeces from animals, or by consumption of foods of animal origin, particularly meat and milk products. The risk of infection can be reduced by avoiding close contact with any animals — including wild, captive and domestic animals — in places where infection is likely to be present. Particular care should be taken to prevent children from approaching and handling animals. Examples of zoonoses are rabies, brucellosis, leptospirosis and certain viral haemorrhagic fevers.

Sexually transmitted diseases

Sexually transmitted diseases are passed from person to person through unsafe sexual practices. The risk of infection can be reduced by avoiding casual and unprotected sexual intercourse, and by use of condoms. Examples of sexually transmitted diseases are hepatitis B, HIV/AIDS and syphilis.

Bloodborne diseases

Bloodborne diseases are transmitted by direct contact with infected blood or other body fluids. The risk of infection can be reduced by avoiding direct contact with blood and body fluids, by avoiding the use of potentially contaminated needles and syringes for injection or any other medical or cosmetic procedure that penetrates the skin (including acupuncture, piercing and tattooing), and by avoiding transfusion of unsafe blood (see Chapter 8). Examples of bloodborne diseases are hepatitis B and C, HIV/AIDS and malaria.

Airborne diseases

Airborne diseases are transmitted from person to person by aerosol and droplets from the nose and mouth. The risk of infection can be reduced by avoiding close contact with people in crowded and enclosed places. Examples of airborne diseases are influenza, meningococcal disease and tuberculosis.

Diseases transmitted from soil

Soil-transmitted diseases include those caused by dormant forms (spores) of infectious agents, which can cause infection by contact with broken skin (minor cuts, scratches, etc.). The risk of infection can be reduced by protecting the skin from direct contact with soil in places where soil-transmitted infections are likely to be present. Examples of bacterial diseases transmitted from soil are anthrax and tetanus. Certain intestinal parasitic infections, such as ascariasis and trichuriasis, are transmitted via soil and infection may result from consumption of soil-contaminated vegetables.

Specific infectious diseases involving potential health risks for travellers

The main infectious diseases to which travellers may be exposed, and precautions for each, are detailed on pages 47–70. Information on malaria, the most important infectious disease threat for travellers, is provided in Chapter 7. Other infectious diseases that affect travellers only rarely are not described in this book. The infectious diseases described in this chapter have been selected on the basis of the following criteria:

— diseases that have a sufficiently high global or regional prevalence to constitute a significant risk for travellers;
— diseases that are severe and life-threatening, even though the risk of exposure may be low for most travellers;
— diseases for which the perceived risk may be much greater than the real risk, and which may therefore cause anxiety to travellers;
— diseases that involve a public health risk due to transmission of infection to others by the infected traveller.

Information about available vaccines and indications for their use by travellers is provided in Chapter 6. Advice concerning the diseases for which vaccination is routinely administered in childhood, i.e. diphtheria, measles, mumps and rubella, pertussis, poliomyelitis and tetanus, and the use of the corresponding vaccines later in life and for travel, is also given in Chapter 6. These diseases are not included in this chapter.

The most common infectious illness to affect travellers, namely travellers' diarrhoea, is covered in Chapter 3. Because travellers' diarrhoea can be caused by many different foodborne and waterborne infectious agents, for which treatment and precautions are essentially the same, the illness is not included with the specific infectious diseases.

Some of the diseases included in this chapter, such as brucellosis, HIV/AIDS, leishmaniasis and tuberculosis, have prolonged and variable incubation periods. Clinical manifestations of these diseases may appear long after the return from travel, so that the link with the travel destination where the infection was acquired may not be readily apparent.

ANTHRAX

Cause	*Bacillus anthracis* bacteria.
Transmission	Cutaneous infection, the most frequent clinical form of anthrax, occurs through contact with contaminated products from infected animals (mainly cattle, goats, sheep), such as leather or woollen goods, or through contact with soil containing anthrax spores.
Nature of the disease	A disease of herbivorous animals that occasionally causes acute infection in humans, usually involving the skin, as a result of contact with contaminated tissues or products from infected animals, or with anthrax spores in soil. Untreated infections may spread to regional lymph nodes and to the bloodstream, and may be fatal.
Geographical distribution	Sporadic cases occur in animals worldwide; there are occasional outbreaks in central Asia.
Risk for travellers	Very low for most travellers.
Prophylaxis	None. (A vaccine is available for people at high risk because of occupational exposure to *B. anthracis*; it is not commercially available in most countries.)
Precautions	Avoid direct contact with soil and with products of animal origin, such as souvenirs made from animal skins.

BRUCELLOSIS

Cause	Several species of *Brucella* bacteria.
Transmission	Brucellosis is primarily a disease of animals. Infection occurs from cattle (*Brucella abortus*), dogs (*B. canis*), pigs (*B. suis*), or sheep and goats (*B. melitensis*), usually by direct contact with infected animals or by consumption of unpasteurized (raw) milk or cheese.
Nature of the disease	A generalized infection with insidious onset, causing continuous or intermittent fever and malaise, which may last for months if not treated adequately. Relapse is common after treatment.
Geographical distribution	Worldwide, in animals. It is most common in developing countries and the Mediterranean region.
Risk for travellers	Low for most travellers. Those visiting rural and agricultural areas may be at greater risk. There is also a risk in places where unpasteurized milk products are sold near tourist centres.
Prophylaxis	None.

47

Precautions	Avoid consumption of unpasteurized milk and milk products and direct contact with animals, particularly cattle, goats and sheep.

CHOLERA

Cause	*Vibrio cholerae* bacteria, serogroups O1 and O139.
Transmission	Infection occurs through ingestion of food or water contaminated directly or indirectly by faeces or vomitus of infected persons. Cholera affects only humans; there is no insect vector or animal reservoir host.
Nature of the disease	An acute enteric disease varying in severity. Most infections are asymptomatic (i.e. do not cause any illness). In mild cases, diarrhoea occurs without other symptoms. In severe cases, there is sudden onset of profuse watery diarrhoea with nausea and vomiting and rapid development of dehydration. In severe untreated cases, death may occur within a few hours due to dehydration leading to circulatory collapse.
Geographical distribution	Cholera occurs mainly in poor countries with inadequate sanitation and lack of clean drinking-water and in war-torn countries where the infrastructure may have broken down. Many developing countries are affected, particularly those in Africa and Asia, and to a lesser extent those in central and south America (see map, page 73).
Risk for travellers	Very low for most travellers, even in countries where cholera epidemics occur. Humanitarian relief workers in disaster areas and refugee camps are at risk.
Prophylaxis	Oral cholera vaccines for use by travellers and those in occupational risk groups are available in some countries (see Chapter 6).
Precautions	As for other diarrhoeal diseases. All precautions should be taken to avoid consumption of potentially contaminated food, drink and drinking-water. Oral rehydration salts should be carried to combat dehydration in case of severe diarrhoea (see Chapter 3).

DENGUE

Cause	The dengue virus—a flavivirus of which there are four serotypes.
Transmission	Dengue is transmitted by the *Aedes aegypti* mosquito, which bites during daylight hours. There is no direct person-to-person transmission. Monkeys act as a reservoir host in south-east Asia and west Africa.
Nature of the disease	Dengue occurs in three main clinical forms: ■ Dengue fever is an acute febrile illness with sudden onset of fever, followed by development of generalized symptoms and sometimes a macular skin rash. It is known as "breakbone fever" because of severe muscular pains. The fever may be biphasic (i.e. two separate episodes or waves of fever). Most patients recover after a few days. ■ Dengue haemorrhagic fever has an acute onset of fever followed by other symptoms resulting from thrombocytopenia, increased vascular permeability and haemorrhagic manifestations.

	■ Dengue shock syndrome supervenes in a small proportion of cases. Severe hypotension develops, requiring urgent medical treatment to correct hypovolaemia. Without appropriate treatment, 40–50% of cases are fatal; with timely therapy, the mortality rate is 1% or less.
Geographical distribution	Dengue is widespread in tropical and subtropical regions of central and south America and south and south-east Asia and also occurs in Africa (see map, page 74); in these regions, dengue is limited to altitudes below 600 metres (2000 feet).
Risk for travellers	There is a significant risk for travellers in areas where dengue is endemic and in areas affected by epidemics of dengue.
Prophylaxis	None.
Precautions	Travellers should take precautions to avoid mosquito bites both during the day and at night in areas where dengue occurs.

FILARIASIS

Cause	The parasitic diseases covered by the term filariasis are caused by nematodes (roundworms) of the family Filarioidea. Diseases in this group include lymphatic filariasis and onchocerciasis (river blindness).
Transmission	Lymphatic filariasis is transmitted through the bite of infected mosquitoes, which inject larval forms of the nematode during a blood meal. Onchocerciasis is transmitted through the bite of infected blackflies.
Nature of the disease	■ Lymphatic filariasis is a chronic parasitic disease in which adult filaria inhabit the lymphatic vessels, discharging microfilaria into the blood stream. Typical manifestations in symptomatic cases include filarial fever, lymphadenitis and retrograde lymphangiitis.
	■ Onchocerciasis is a chronic parasitic disease occurring mainly in sub-Saharan west Africa in which adult worms are found in fibrous nodules under the skin. They discharge microfilaria, which migrate through the skin causing dermatitis, and reach the eye causing damage that results in blindness.
Geographical distribution	Lymphatic filariasis occurs throughout sub-Saharan Africa and in much of south-east Asia. Onchocerciasis occurs mainly in western and central Africa, also in central and south America.
Risk for travellers	Generally low, unless travel involves extensive exposure to the vectors in endemic areas.
Prophylaxis	None.
Precautions	Avoid exposure to the bites of mosquitoes and/or blackflies in endemic areas.

GIARDIASIS

Cause	The protozoan parasite *Giardia lamblia*.

Transmission	Infection usually occurs through ingestion of Giardia cysts in water (including both unfiltered drinking-water and recreational waters) contaminated by the faeces of infected humans or animals.
Nature of the disease	Many infections are asymptomatic. When symptoms occur, they are mainly intestinal, characterized by anorexia, chronic diarrhoea, abdominal cramps, bloating, frequent loose greasy stools, fatigue and weight loss.
Geographical distribution	Worldwide.
Risk for travellers	Significant risk for travellers in contact with recreational waters used by wildlife or with unfiltered water in swimming pools.
Prophylaxis	None.
Precautions	Avoid ingesting any potentially contaminated (i.e. unfiltered) drinking-water or recreational water.

HAEMOPHILUS MENINGITIS

Cause	*Haemophilus influenzae* type b (Hib) bacteria.
Transmission	Direct contact with an infected person (usually children).
Nature of the disease	Hib causes meningitis in infants and young children; it may also cause epiglottitis, osteomyelitis, pneumonia, sepsis and septic arthritis.
Geographical distribution	Worldwide. Hib disease is most common in countries where vaccination against Hib is not practised. It has almost disappeared in countries where routine childhood vaccination is carried out.
Risk for travellers	A risk for unvaccinated children visiting countries where Hib vaccination is not practised and where infection is therefore likely to be more common.
Prophylaxis	Vaccination of children (see Chapter 6).
Precautions	None.

HAEMORRHAGIC FEVERS

Haemorrhagic fevers are viral infections; important examples are Crimean–Congo haemorrhagic fever (CCHF), dengue, Ebola and Marburg haemorrhagic fevers, Lassa fever, Rift Valley fever (RVF) and yellow fever.

Dengue and yellow fever are described separately.

Cause	Viruses belonging to several families. Most haemorrhagic fevers, including dengue and yellow fever, are caused by flaviviruses; Ebola and Marburg are caused by filoviruses, CCHF by a bunyavirus, Lassa fever by an arenavirus, and RVF by a phlebovirus.
Transmission	Most viruses that cause haemorrhagic fevers are transmitted by mosquitoes. However, no insect vector has so far been identified for Ebola or Marburg viruses: these viruses are acquired by direct contact with the body fluids or secretions of infected patients. CCHF is transmitted by ticks. Lassa fever virus is carried by rodents and transmitted by excreta, either as aerosol

	or by direct contact. RVF can be acquired either by mosquito bite or by direct contact with blood or tissues of infected animals (mainly sheep), including consumption of unpasteurized milk.
Nature of the diseases	The haemorrhagic fevers are severe acute viral infections, usually with sudden onset of fever, malaise, headache and myalgia followed by pharyngitis, vomiting, diarrhoea, skin rash and haemorrhagic manifestations. The outcome is fatal in a high proportion of cases (over 50%).
Geographical distribution	Diseases in this group occur widely in tropical and subtropical regions. Ebola and Marburg haemorrhagic fevers and Lassa fever occur in sub-Saharan Africa. CCHF occurs in the steppe regions of central Asia and in central Europe, as well as in tropical and southern Africa. RVF occurs in Africa and has recently spread to Saudi Arabia. Other viral haemorrhagic fevers occur in central and south America.
Risk for travellers	Very low for most travellers. However, travellers visiting rural or forest areas may be exposed to infection.
Prophylaxis	None (except for yellow fever).
Precautions	Avoid exposure to mosquitoes and ticks and contact with rodents.

HANTAVIRUS DISEASES

Hantavirus diseases are viral infections; important examples are haemorrhagic fever with renal syndrome (HFRS) and hantavirus pulmonary syndrome (HPS).

Cause	Hantaviruses, which belong to the family of bunyaviruses.
Transmission	Hantaviruses are carried by various species of rodents. Infection occurs through direct contact with the faeces, saliva or urine of infected rodents or by inhalation of the virus by aerosol transmission from rodent excreta.
Nature of the diseases	Acute viral diseases in which vascular endothelium is damaged, leading to increased vascular permeability, hypotension, haemorrhagic manifestations and shock. Impaired renal function with oliguria is characteristic of HFRS. Respiratory distress due to pulmonary oedema occurs in HPS. The outcome is fatal in up to 15% of HFRS cases and up to 50% of HPS cases.
Geographical distribution	Worldwide, in rodents.
Risk for travellers	Very low for most travellers. However, travellers may be at risk in any environment where rodents are present in large numbers and contact may occur.
Prophylaxis	None.
Precautions	Avoid exposure to rodents and their excreta. Adventure travellers, backpackers, campers and travellers with occupational exposure to rodents in areas endemic for hantaviruses should take precautions to exclude rodents from tents or other accommodation and to protect all food from contamination by rodents.

HEPATITIS A

Cause	Hepatitis A virus, a member of the picornavirus family.
Transmission	The virus is acquired directly from infected persons by the faecal–oral route or by close contact, or by consumption of contaminated food or drinking-water. There is no insect vector or animal reservoir (although some non-human primates are sometimes infected).
Nature of the disease	An acute viral hepatitis with abrupt onset of fever, malaise, nausea and abdominal discomfort, followed by the development of jaundice a few days later. Infection in very young children is usually mild or asymptomatic; older children are at risk of symptomatic disease. The disease is more severe in adults, with illness lasting several weeks and recovery taking several months; case-fatality is greater than 2% for those over 40 years of age and 4% for those over 60.
Geographical distribution	Worldwide, but most common where sanitary conditions are poor and the safety of drinking-water is not well controlled (see map, page 75).
Risk for travellers	Non-immune travellers to developing countries are at significant risk of infection. The risk is particularly high for travellers exposed to poor conditions of hygiene, sanitation and drinking-water control.
Prophylaxis	Vaccination (see Chapter 6).
Precautions	Travellers who are non-immune to hepatitis A (i.e. have never had the disease and have not been vaccinated) should take particular care to avoid potentially contaminated food and water.

HEPATITIS B

Cause	Hepatitis B virus (HBV), belonging to the Hepadnaviridae.
Transmission	Infection is transmitted from person to person by contact with infected body fluids. Sexual contact is an important mode of transmission, but infection is also transmitted by transfusion of contaminated blood or blood products, or by use of contaminated needles or syringes for injections. There is also a potential risk of transmission through other skin-penetrating procedures including acupuncture, piercing and tattooing. Perinatal transmission may occur from mother to baby. There is no insect vector or animal reservoir.
Nature of the disease	Many HBV infections are asymptomatic or cause mild symptoms, which are often unrecognized in adults. When clinical hepatitis results from infection, it has a gradual onset, with anorexia, abdominal discomfort, nausea, vomiting, arthralgia and rash, followed by the development of jaundice in some cases. In adults, about 1% of cases are fatal. Chronic HBV infection persists in a proportion of adults, some of whom later develop cirrhosis and/or liver cancer.
Geographical distribution	Worldwide, but with differing levels of endemicity. In north America, Australia, northern and western Europe and New Zealand, prevalence of chronic HBV infection is relatively low (less than 2% of the general population) (see map, page 76).

Risk for travellers	Negligible for those vaccinated against hepatitis B. Unvaccinated travellers are at risk if they have unprotected sex or use contaminated needles or syringes for injection, acupuncture, piercing or tattooing. An accident or medical emergency requiring blood transfusion may result in infection if the blood has not been screened for HBV. Travellers engaged in humanitarian relief activities may be exposed to infected blood or other body fluids in health care settings (see box, page 56).
Prophylaxis	Vaccination (see Chapter 6).
Precautions	Adopt safe sexual practices and avoid the use of any potentially contaminated instruments for injection or other skin-piercing activity.

HEPATITIS C

Cause	Hepatitis C virus (HCV), which is a flavivirus.
Transmission	The virus is acquired through person-to-person transmission by parenteral routes. Before screening for HCV became available, infection was mainly transmitted by transfusion of contaminated blood or blood products. Nowadays transmission frequently occurs through use of contaminated needles, syringes and other instruments used for injections and other skin-piercing procedures. Sexual transmission of hepatitis C occurs rarely. There is no insect vector or animal reservoir for HCV.
Nature of the disease	Most HCV infections are asymptomatic. In cases where infection leads to clinical hepatitis, the onset of symptoms is usually gradual, with anorexia, abdominal discomfort, nausea and vomiting, followed by the development of jaundice in some cases (less commonly than in hepatitis B). Most clinically affected patients will develop a long-lasting chronic infection, which may lead to cirrhosis and/or liver cancer.
Geographical distribution	Worldwide, with regional differences in levels of prevalence, as shown on the map (page 77).
Risk for travellers	Travellers are at risk if they practise unsafe behaviour involving the use of contaminated needles or syringes for injection, acupuncture, piercing or tattooing. An accident or medical emergency requiring blood transfusion (see box, page 56) may result in infection if the blood has not been screened for HCV. Travellers engaged in humanitarian relief activities may be exposed to infected blood or other body fluids in health care settings.
Prophylaxis	None.
Precautions	Adopt safe sexual practices and avoid the use of any potentially contaminated instruments for injection or other skin-piercing activity.

HEPATITIS E

Cause	Hepatitis E virus, which has not yet been definitively classified but probably belongs to the Caliciviridae.
Transmission	Hepatitis E is a waterborne disease usually acquired from contaminated drinking-water. Direct faecal–oral transmission from person to person is

	also possible. There is no insect vector. It is suspected, but not proved, that hepatitis E may have a domestic animal reservoir host, such as pigs.
Nature of the disease	The clinical features and course of the disease are generally similar to those of hepatitis A. As with hepatitis A, there is no chronic phase. Young adults are most commonly affected. In pregnant women there is an important difference between hepatitis E and hepatitis A: during the third trimester of pregnancy, hepatitis E takes a much more severe form with a case-fatality rate reaching 20%.
Geographical distribution	Worldwide. Most cases, both sporadic and epidemic, occur in countries with poor standards of hygiene and sanitation.
Risk for travellers	Travellers to developing countries may be at risk when exposed to poor conditions of sanitation and drinking-water control.
Prophylaxis	None.
Precautions	Travellers should follow the general conditions for avoiding potentially contaminated food and drinking-water (see Chapter 3).

HIV/AIDS AND OTHER SEXUALLY TRANSMITTED INFECTIONS

The most important sexually transmitted diseases and infectious agents are:

HIV/AIDS	human immunodeficiency virus
hepatitis B	hepatitis B virus
syphilis	*Treponema pallidum*
gonorrhoea	*Neisseria gonorrhoeae*
chlamydial infections	*Chlamydia trachomatis*
trichomoniasis	*Trichomonas vaginalis*
chancroid	*Haemophilus ducreyi*
genital herpes	herpes simplex virus (human (alpha) herpesvirus 1)
genital warts	human papillomavirus

Travel restrictions

Some countries have adopted entry and visa restrictions for people with HIV/AIDS. Travellers who are infected with HIV should consult their personal physician for a detailed assessment and advice before travel. WHO has taken the position that there is no public health justification for entry restrictions that discriminate solely on the basis of a person's HIV status.

Transmission	Infection occurs during unprotected sexual intercourse. Hepatitis B, HIV and syphilis may also be transmitted in contaminated blood and blood products, by contaminated syringes and needles used for injection, and potentially by unsterilized instruments used for acupuncture, piercing and tattooing.
Nature of the diseases	Most of the clinical manifestations are included in the following syndromes: genital ulcer, pelvic inflammatory disease, urethral discharge and vaginal discharge. However, many infections are asymptomatic.
	Sexually transmitted infections are a major cause of acute illness, infertility, long-term disability and death, with severe medical and psychological consequences for millions of men, women and children.

	Apart from being serious diseases in their own right, sexually transmitted infections increase the risk of HIV infection. The presence of an untreated disease (ulcerative or non-ulcerative) can increase by a factor of up to 10 the risk of becoming infected with HIV and transmitting the infection. On the other hand, early diagnosis and improved management of other sexually transmitted infections can reduce the incidence of HIV infection by up to 40%. Prevention and treatment of all sexually transmitted infections are therefore important for the prevention of HIV infection.
Geographical distribution	Worldwide (see map, page 78). The regional differences in the prevalence of HIV infection are shown on the map (page 78). Sexually transmitted infections have been known since ancient times; they remain a major public health problem, which was compounded by the appearance of HIV/AIDS around 1980. An estimated 340 million episodes of curable sexually transmitted infections (chlamydial infections, gonorrhoea, syphilis, trichomoniasis) occur throughout the world every year. Viral infections, which are more difficult to treat, are also very common in many populations. Genital herpes is becoming a major cause of genital ulcer, and subtypes of the human papillomavirus are associated with cervical cancer.
Risk for travellers	For some travellers there may be an increased risk of infection. Lack of information about risk and preventive measures and the fact that travel and tourism enhance the probability of having sex with casual partners increase the risk of exposure to sexually transmitted infections. In some developed countries, a large proportion of sexually transmitted infections now occur as a result of unprotected sexual intercourse during international travel. In addition to transmission through sexual intercourse (both heterosexual and homosexual—anal, vaginal or oral), most of these infections can be passed on from an infected mother to her unborn or newborn baby. Hepatitis B, HIV and syphilis are also transmitted through transfusion of contaminated blood or blood products and the use of contaminated needles (see box, page 56). There is no risk of acquiring any sexually transmitted infection from casual day-to-day contact at home, at work or socially. People run no risk of infection when sharing any means of communal transport (e.g. aircraft, boat, bus, car, train) with infected individuals. There is no evidence that HIV or other sexually transmitted infections can be acquired from insect bites.
Prophylaxis	Vaccination against hepatitis B (see Chapter 6). No prophylaxis is available for any of the other sexually transmitted diseases.
Precautions	Male or female condoms, when properly used, have proved to be effective in preventing the transmission of HIV and other sexually transmitted infections, and for reducing the risk of unwanted pregnancy. Latex rubber condoms are relatively inexpensive, are highly reliable and have virtually no side-effects. The transmission of HIV and other infections during sexual intercourse can be effectively prevented when high-quality condoms are used correctly and consistently. Studies on serodiscordant couples (only one of whom is HIV-positive) have shown that, with regular sexual intercourse over a period of two years, partners who consistently use condoms have a near-zero risk of HIV infection.

Accidental exposure to blood or other body fluids

Accidental exposure to blood or other body fluids may occur in health care settings, during natural or manmade disasters, or as a result of accidents or acts of violence. This may lead to infection by bloodborne pathogens, particularly hepatitis B and C viruses and HIV. The average risk of seroconversion to HIV after a single percutaneous exposure to HIV-infected blood is 0.3%; the risk for hepatitis C is 3% and for hepatitis B it is 10–30%.

Accidental exposure to potentially infected blood or other body fluids is a medical emergency. The following measures should be taken without delay.

Percutaneous exposure

In the case of injury with equipment contaminated with blood or contact of broken skin with blood or other body fluids, allow the wound to bleed freely; wash the wound and surrounding skin immediately with soap and water and rinse. Disinfect the wound and surrounding skin with a suitable disinfectant such as:

— povidone iodine 2.5% for 5 minutes, or

— alcohol 70% for 3 minutes.

Exposure of the eyes or mucous membranes

Rinse the exposed area immediately with an isotonic saline solution for 10 minutes. In the case of contamination of mucosa of the eye, disinfect with chlorhexidine–cetrimide 0.05%, 3 drops given twice at an interval of 10 minutes. If neither saline nor disinfectant is available, use clean water.

In all cases, a physician should be contacted immediately.

Under certain conditions, the use of a combination of antiretroviral drugs is the recommended prophylactic intervention to prevent transmission of HIV after accidental exposure to infected blood or other body fluids. The decision to provide this treatment depends on a number of factors, including the HIV status of the source individual, the nature of the body fluid involved, the severity of exposure and the period between the exposure and the beginning of treatment (which should never be more than 48 hours). Repatriation should be carried out as soon as possible.

If HIV and hepatitis B and C testing has been done, subsequent tests will be necessary 6 weeks following exposure and 6 months following exposure. People who test positive at these stages should be offered psychological support.

After accidental exposure, the exposed individual should not have unprotected sexual intercourse until the 6-months post-exposure tests confirm that he/she is not seropositive. Women should avoid becoming pregnant during this period.

A man should always use a condom during sexual intercourse, each time, from start to finish, and a woman should make sure that her partner uses one. A woman can also protect herself from sexually transmitted infections by using a female condom—essentially, a vaginal pouch—which is now commercially available in some countries.

It is essential to avoid injecting drugs for non-medical purposes, and particularly to avoid any type of needle-sharing to reduce the risk of acquiring hepatitis, HIV, syphilis and other infections from contaminated needles and blood.

Medical injections using unsterilized equipment are also a possible source of infection. If an injection is essential, the traveller should try to ensure that the needles and syringes come from a sterile package or have been sterilized properly by steam or boiling water for 20 minutes.

Patients under medical care who require frequent injections, e.g. diabetics, should carry sufficient sterile needles and syringes for the duration of their trip and a doctor's authorization for their use.

Unsterile dental and surgical instruments, needles used in acupuncture and tattooing, ear-piercing devices, and other skin-piercing instruments can likewise transmit infection and should be avoided.

Treatment	Travellers with signs or symptoms of a sexually transmitted disease should cease all sexual activity and seek medical care immediately. The absence of symptoms does not guarantee absence of infection, and travellers exposed to unprotected sex should be tested for infection on returning home. HIV testing should always be voluntary and with counselling.

The sexually transmitted infections caused by bacteria, e.g. chancroid, chlamydia, gonorrhoea and syphilis, can be treated successfully, but there is no single antimicrobial that is effective against more than one or two of them. Moreover, throughout the world, many of these bacteria are showing increased resistance to penicillin and other antimicrobials.

Treatment for sexually transmitted viral infections, e.g. hepatitis B, genital herpes and genital warts, is unsatisfactory due to lack of specific medication, and cure is difficult to achieve. The same is true of HIV infection, which in its late stage causes AIDS and is thought to be invariably fatal. Antiretroviral drugs cannot completely eradicate the HIV virus; treatment is expensive and complex and most countries have only a few centres that are able to provide it.

INFLUENZA

Cause	Influenza viruses of types A, B and C; type A occurs in two subtypes (H1N1 and H3N2). Type A viruses cause most of the widespread influenza epidemics; type B viruses generally cause regional outbreaks, and type C are of minor significance for humans.

Influenza viruses evolve rapidly, changing their antigenic characteristics, so that vaccines need to be modified each year to be effective against currently circulating influenza strains.

	Other types and subtypes of influenza viruses occur in animals and birds; transmission and reassortment between species may give rise to new subtypes able to infect humans.
Transmission	Airborne transmission of influenza viruses occurs particularly in crowded enclosed spaces. Transmission also occurs by direct contact with droplets disseminated by unprotected coughs and sneezes and contamination of the hands.
Nature of the disease	An acute respiratory infection of varying severity, ranging from asymptomatic infection to fatal disease. Initial symptoms include fever with rapid onset, sore throat, cough and chills, often accompanied by headache, coryza, myalgia and prostration. Influenza may be complicated by viral or more often bacterial pneumonia. Illness tends to be most severe in the elderly and in young children. Death resulting from influenza occurs mainly in the elderly and in individuals with pre-existing chronic diseases.
Geographical distribution	Worldwide. In temperate regions, influenza is a seasonal disease occurring in winter: it affects the northern hemisphere from November to March and the southern hemisphere from April to September. In tropical areas there is no clear seasonal pattern, and influenza may occur at any time of the year.
Risk for travellers	Travellers, like local residents, are at risk in any country during the influenza season. Travellers visiting countries in the opposite hemisphere during the influenza season are at special risk, particularly if they have not built up some degree of immunity through regular vaccination. The elderly, people with pre-existing chronic diseases and young children are most susceptible.
Prophylaxis	Vaccination before the start of the influenza season. However, vaccine for visitors to the opposite hemisphere is unlikely to be obtainable before arrival at the travel destination (see Chapter 6).
	For travellers in the highest risk groups for severe and complicated influenza who have not been or cannot be vaccinated, the prophylactic use of antiviral drugs such as zanamivir and oseltamivir is indicated in countries where they are available. Amantidine and rimantidine may also be considered.
Precautions	Whenever possible, avoid crowded enclosed spaces and close contact with people suffering from acute respiratory infections.

JAPANESE ENCEPHALITIS

Cause	Japanese encephalitis (JE) virus, which is a flavivirus.
Transmission	The virus is transmitted by various mosquitoes of the genus *Culex*. It infects pigs and various wild birds as well as humans. Mosquitoes become infective after feeding on viraemic pigs or birds.
Nature of the disease	Most infections are asymptomatic. In symptomatic cases, severity varies; mild infections are characterized by febrile headache or aseptic meningitis. Severe cases have a rapid onset and progression, with headache, high fever and meningeal signs. There may be neurological sequelae after recovery. Approximately 50% of severe clinical cases have a fatal outcome.

Geographical distribution	JE occurs in a number of countries in Asia (see map, page 79) and occasionally in northern Queensland, Australia.
Risk for travellers	Low for most travellers. Visitors to rural and agricultural areas in endemic countries may be at risk, particularly during epidemics of JE.
Prophylaxis	Vaccination, if justified by likelihood of exposure (see Chapter 6).
Precautions	Avoid mosquito bites (see Chapter 3).

LEGIONELLOSIS

Cause	Various species of Legionella bacteria, frequently Legionella pneumophila, serogroup I.
Transmission	Infection results from inhalation of contaminated water sprays or mists. The bacteria live in water and colonize hot-water systems at temperatures of 20–50 °C (optimal 35–46 °C). They contaminate air-conditioning cooling towers, hot-water systems, humidifiers, whirlpool spas and other water-containing devices. There is no direct person-to-person transmission.
Nature of the disease	Legionellosis occurs in two distinct clinical forms:
	■ Legionnaires disease is an acute bacterial pneumonia with rapid onset of anorexia, malaise, myalgia, headache and rapidly rising fever, progressing to pneumonia, which may lead to respiratory failure and death.
	■ Pontiac fever is an influenza-like illness with spontaneous recovery after 2–5 days.
	Susceptibility to legionellosis increases with age, especially among smokers and people with pre-existing chronic lung disease or other immuno-compromising conditions.
Geographical distribution	Worldwide.
Risk for travellers	Generally low. Outbreaks occasionally occur through dissemination of infection by contaminated water or air-conditioning systems in hotels and other facilities used by visitors.
Prophylaxis	None. Prevention of infection depends on regular cleaning and disinfection of possible sources.
Precautions	None.

LEISHMANIASIS (including espundia or oriental sore, and kala-azar)

Cause	Several species of the protozoan parasite Leishmania.
Transmission	Infection is transmitted by the bite of female phlebotomine sandflies. Dogs, rodents and other mammals are reservoir hosts for leishmaniasis. Sandflies acquire the parasites by biting infected humans or animals. Transmission from person to person by injected blood or contaminated syringes and needles is also possible.

59

Nature of the disease	Leishmaniasis occurs in two main forms:
	■ Cutaneous and mucosal leishmaniasis (espundia) cause skin sores and chronic ulcers of the mucosae. Cutaneous leishmaniasis is a chronic, progressive, disabling and often mutilating disease.
	■ Visceral leishmaniasis (kala-azar) affects the bone marrow, liver, spleen, lymph nodes and other internal organs. It is usually fatal if untreated.
Geographical distribution	Many countries in tropical and subtropical regions, including Africa, parts of central and south America, Asia, southern Europe and the eastern Mediterranean. Over 90% of all cases of visceral leishmaniasis occur in Bangladesh, Brazil, India, Nepal and Sudan. More than 90% of all cases of cutaneous leishmaniasis occur in Afghanistan, Algeria, Brazil, the Islamic Republic of Iran, Saudi Arabia and the Syrian Arab Republic.
Risk for travellers	Generally low. Visitors to rural and forested areas in endemic countries are at risk.
Prophylaxis	None.
Precautions	Avoid sandfly bites, particularly after sunset, by using repellents and insecticide-impregnated bednets. The bite leaves a non-swollen red ring, which can alert the traveller to its origin.

LEPTOSPIROSIS (including Weil disease)

Cause	Various spirochaetes of the genus *Leptospira*.
Transmission	Infection occurs through contact between the skin (particularly skin abrasions) or mucous membranes and water, wet soil or vegetation contaminated by the urine of infected animals, notably rats. Occasionally infection may result from direct contact with urine or tissues of infected animals, or from consumption of food contaminated by the urine of infected rats.
Nature of the disease	Leptospiral infections take many different clinical forms, usually with sudden onset of fever, headache, myalgia, chills, conjunctival suffusion and skin rash. The disease may progress to meningitis, haemolytic anaemia, jaundice, haemorrhagic manifestations and other complications, including hepatorenal failure.
Geographical distribution	Worldwide. Most common in tropical countries.
Risk for travellers	Low for most travellers. There is occupational risk for farmers in paddy rice and sugar cane production. Visitors to rural areas and in contact with water in canals, lakes and rivers may be exposed to infection. There is increased risk after recent floods. The risk may be greater for those who practise canoeing, kayaking or other activities in water.
Prophylaxis	None. Vaccine against local strains is available for workers where the disease is an occupational hazard but is not commercially available in most countries.
Precautions	Avoid swimming or wading in potentially contaminated waters including canals, ponds, rivers, streams and swamps. Avoid all direct or indirect contact with rodents.

LISTERIOSIS

Cause	The bacterium *Listeria monocytogenes*.
Transmission	Listeriosis affects a variety of animals. Foodborne infection in humans occurs through the consumption of contaminated foods, particularly unpasteurized milk, soft cheeses, vegetables and prepared meat products such as pâté. Listeriosis multiplies readily in refrigerated foods that have been contaminated, unlike most foodborne pathogens. Transmission can also occur from mother to fetus or from mother to child during birth.
Nature of the disease	Listeriosis causes meningoencephalitis and/or septicaemia in adults and newborn infants. In pregnant women, it causes fever and abortion. Newborn infants, pregnant women, the elderly and immunocompromised individuals are particularly susceptible to listeriosis. In others, the disease may be limited to a mild acute febrile episode. In pregnant women, transmission of infection to the fetus may lead to stillbirth, septicaemia at birth or neonatal meningitis.
Geographical distribution	Worldwide, with sporadic incidence.
Risk for travellers	Generally low. Risk is increased by consumption of unpasteurized milk and milk products and prepared meat products.
Prophylaxis	None.
Precautions	Avoid consumption of unpasteurized milk and milk products. Pregnant women and immunocompromised individuals should take stringent precautions to avoid infection by listeriosis and other foodborne pathogens (see Chapter 3).

LYME BORRELIOSIS (Lyme disease)

Cause	The spirochaete *Borrelia burgdorferi*, of which there are several different serotypes.
Transmission	Infection occurs through the bite of infected ticks, both adults and nymphs, of the genus *Ixodes*. Most human infections result from bites by nymphs. Many species of mammals can be infected, and deer act as an important reservoir.
Nature of the disease	The disease usually has its onset in summer. Early skin lesions have an expanding ring form, often with a central clear zone. Fever, chills, myalgia and headache are common. Meningeal involvement may follow. Central nervous system and other complications may occur weeks or months after the onset of illness. Arthritis may develop up to 2 years after onset.
Geographical distribution	There are endemic foci of Lyme borreliosis in forested areas of Asia, north-western, central and eastern Europe, and the USA.
Risk for travellers	Generally low. Visitors to rural areas in endemic regions, particularly campers and hikers, are at risk.
Prophylaxis	A vaccine available in the USA provides protection against the specific serotype endemic in the USA (see Chapter 6).

Precautions	Avoid tick-infested areas and exposure to ticks (see Chapter 3). If a bite occurs, remove the tick as soon as possible.

MALARIA

See Chapter 7 and map, page 80.

MENINGOCOCCAL DISEASE

Cause	The bacterium *Neisseria meningitidis*, of which 12 serotypes are known. Most cases of meningococcal disease are caused by serogroups A, B and C; less commonly, infection is caused by serogroups Y and W-135. Epidemics in Africa are usually caused by *N. meningitidis* type A.
Transmission	Transmission occurs by direct person-to-person contact, including aerosol transmission and respiratory droplets from the nose and pharynx of infected persons, patients or asymptomatic carriers. There is no animal reservoir or insect vector.
Nature of the disease	Most infections do not cause clinical disease. Many infected people become asymptomatic carriers of the bacteria and serve as a reservoir and source of infection for others. In general, susceptibility to meningococcal disease decreases with age, although there is a small increase in risk in adolescents and young adults. Meningococcal meningitis has a sudden onset of intense headache, fever, nausea, vomiting, photophobia and stiff neck, plus various neurological signs. The disease is fatal in 5–10% of cases even with prompt antimicrobial treatment in good health care facilities; among individuals who survive, up to 20% have permanent neurological sequelae. Meningococcal septicaemia, in which there is rapid dissemination of bacteria in the bloodstream, is a less common form of meningococcal disease, characterized by circulatory collapse, haemorrhagic skin rash and high fatality rate.
Geographical distribution	Sporadic cases are found worldwide. In temperate zones, most cases occur in the winter months. Localized outbreaks occur in enclosed crowded spaces (e.g. dormitories, military barracks). In sub-Saharan Africa, in a zone stretching across the continent from Senegal to Ethiopia (the African "meningitis belt"), large outbreaks and epidemics take place during the dry season (November–June).
Risk for travellers	Generally low. However, the risk is considerable if travellers are in crowded conditions or take part in large population movements such as pilgrimages in the Sahel meningitis belt. Localized outbreaks occasionally occur among travellers (usually young adults) in camps or dormitories. See also Chapter 6 for specific risks for travellers.
Prophylaxis	Vaccination is available for *N. meningitidis* types A, C, Y and W-135 (see Chapter 6).
Precautions	Avoid overcrowding in confined spaces. Following close contact with a person suffering from meningococcal disease, medical advice should be sought regarding chemoprophylaxis.

PLAGUE

Cause	The plague bacillus, *Yersinia pestis*.
Transmission	Plague is a zoonotic disease affecting rodents and transmitted by fleas from rats to other animals and to humans. Direct person-to-person transmission does not occur except in the case of pneumonic plague, when respiratory droplets may transfer the infection from the patient to others in close contact.
Nature of the disease	Plague occurs in three main clinical forms: ■ Bubonic plague is the form that usually results from the bite of infected fleas. Lymphadenitis develops in the drainage lymph nodes, with the regional lymph nodes most commonly affected. Swelling, pain and suppuration of the lymph nodes produces the characteristic plague buboes. ■ Septicaemic plague may develop from bubonic plague or occur in the absence of lymphadenitis. Dissemination of the infection in the bloodstream results in meningitis, endotoxic shock and disseminated intravascular coagulation. ■ Pneumonic plague may result from secondary infection of the lungs following dissemination of plague bacilli from other body sites. It produces severe pneumonia. Direct infection of others may result from transfer of infection by respiratory droplets, causing primary pulmonary plague in the recipients. Without prompt and effective treatment, 50–60% of cases of bubonic plague are fatal, while untreated septicaemic and pneumonic plague are invariably fatal.
Geographical distribution	There are natural foci of plague infection of rats in many parts of the world. Wild rodent plague is present in central, eastern and southern Africa, south America, the western part of north America and in large areas of Asia. In some areas, contact between wild and domestic rats is common, resulting in sporadic cases of human plague and occasional outbreaks.
Risk for travellers	Generally low. However, travellers in rural areas of plague-endemic regions may be at risk, particularly if camping or hunting or if contact with rodents takes place.
Prophylaxis	A vaccine effective against bubonic plague is available exclusively for persons with a high occupational exposure to plague; it is not commercially available in most countries.
Precautions	Avoid any contact with live or dead rodents.

RABIES

Cause	The rabies virus, a rhabdovirus of the genus *Lyssavirus*.
Transmission	Rabies is a zoonotic disease affecting a wide range of domestic and wild animals, including bats. Infection of humans usually occurs through the bite of an infected animal. The virus is present in the saliva. Any other contact involving penetration of the skin occurring in an area where rabies is present should be treated with caution. In developing countries

Rabies post-exposure treatment

In a rabies-endemic area, the circumstances of an animal bite, other contact with the animal, and the animal's behaviour and appearance may suggest that it is rabid. In such situations, medical advice should be obtained immediately.

Post-exposure treatment to prevent the establishment of rabies infection involves first-aid treatment of the wound followed by administration of rabies vaccine and antirabies immunoglobulin in the case of class 3 exposure. The administration of vaccine, and immunoglobulin if required, must be carried out, or directly supervised, by a physician.

Post-exposure treatment depends on the type of contact with the confirmed or suspect rabid animal, as follows:

Type of contact (class of exposure)	Recommended treatment
1. Touching or feeding animals Licks on the skin	None
2. Nibbling unbroken skin Minor scratches without bleeding Licks on broken skin	Administer vaccine immediately[1]
3. Single or multiple bites or scratches with skin penetration Contamination of mucous membrane by saliva from licking	Administer antirabies immunoglobulin and vaccine immediately

First-aid treatment

Since elimination of the rabies virus at the site of infection by chemical or physical means is the most effective mechanism of protection, immediate vigorous washing and flushing with soap or detergent and water, or water alone, is imperative. Following washing, apply either ethanol (70%) or tincture or aqueous solution of iodine or povidone iodine.

Specific treatment

Antirabies immunoglobulin (RIG) is applied by instillation into the depth of the wound and by infiltration of the surrounding tissues. As much as possible of the total RIG volume required should be instilled into the wound. Vaccine[2] is applied by intradermal or intra-muscular injection in schedules requiring several doses (4 or 5 doses by intramuscular injection, depending on the vaccine used), with the first dose being administered as soon as possible after exposure and the last dose within 28 days for intramuscular or 90 days for intradermal vaccination.

Patients who have been vaccinated prophylactically against rabies with a full course of cell-culture or duck-embryo vaccine can be given a shorter course of post-exposure treatment with fewer doses; they do not require RIG. Urgent post-exposure treatment remains essential whether or not patients have been previously vaccinated.

---

[1] Treatment can be stopped if the suspect animal is shown by appropriate laboratory examination to be free of rabies or, in the case of domestic dogs and cats, if the animal remains healthy throughout a 10-day observation period.

[2] Modern rabies vaccines, made from cell-culture or duck-embryo-derived rabies virus which is then purified and inactivated, are replacing the older vaccines produced in brain tissue.

	transmission is usually from dogs. Person-to-person transmission has not been documented.
Nature of the disease	An acute viral encephalomyelitis, which is almost invariably fatal. The initial signs include a sense of apprehension, headache, fever, malaise and sensory changes around the site of the animal bite. Excitability, hallucinations and aerophobia are common, followed in some cases by fear of water (hydrophobia) due to spasms of the swallowing muscles, progressing to delirium, convulsions and death a few days after onset. A less common form, paralytic rabies, is characterized by loss of sensation, weakness, pain and paralysis.
Geographical distribution	Rabies is present in animals in many countries worldwide (see map, page 82). Most cases of human infection occur in developing countries.
Risk for travellers	In rabies-endemic areas, travellers may be at risk if there is contact with both wild and domestic animals, including dogs and cats.
Prophylaxis	Vaccination for travellers with a foreseeable significant risk of exposure to rabies or travelling to a hyperendemic area where modern rabies vaccine may not be available (see Chapter 6).
Precautions	Avoid contact with wild animals and stray domestic animals, particularly dogs and cats, in rabies-endemic areas. If bitten by an animal that is potentially infected with rabies, or after other suspect contact, immediately clean the wound thoroughly with disinfectant or with soap or detergent and water. Medical assistance should be sought immediately (see box, page 64).
	The vaccination status of the animal involved should not be a criterion for withholding post-exposure treatment, unless the vaccination has been thoroughly documented and vaccine of known potency has been used. In the case of domestic animals, the suspect animal should be kept under observation for a period of 10 days.

SCHISTOSOMIASIS (bilharziasis)

Cause	Several species of parasitic blood flukes (trematodes), of which the most important are *Schistosoma mansoni*, *S. japonicum* and *S. haematobium*.
Transmission	Infection occurs in fresh water containing larval forms (cercariae) of schistosomes, which develop in snails. The free-swimming larvae penetrate the skin of individuals swimming or wading in water. Snails become infected as a result of excretion of eggs in human urine or faeces.
Nature of the disease	Chronic conditions in which adult flukes live for many years in the veins (mesenteric or vesical) of the host where they produce eggs, which cause damage to the organs in which they are deposited. The symptoms depend on the main target organs affected by the different species, with *S. mansoni* and *S. japonicum* causing hepatic and intestinal signs and *S. haematobium* causing urinary dysfunction. The larvae of some schistosomes of birds and other animals may penetrate human skin and cause a self-limiting dermatitis, "swimmers itch". These larvae are unable to develop in humans.

Geographical distribution	*S. mansoni* occurs in many countries of sub-Saharan Africa, in the Arabian peninsula, and in Brazil, Suriname and Venezuela. *S. japonicum* is found in China, in parts of Indonesia, and in the Philippines (but no longer in Japan). *S. haematobium* is present in sub-Saharan Africa and in eastern Mediterranean areas.
Risk for travellers	In endemic areas, travellers are at risk while swimming or wading in fresh water.
Prophylaxis	None.
Precautions	Avoid direct contact (swimming or wading) with potentially contaminated fresh water in endemic areas. In case of accidental exposure, dry the skin vigorously to reduce penetration by cercariae. Avoid drinking, washing, or washing clothing in water that may contain cercariae. Water can be treated to remove or inactivate cercariae by paper filtering or use of iodine or chlorine.

TICK-BORNE ENCEPHALITIS (spring–summer encephalitis)

Cause	The tick-borne encephalitis (TBE) virus, which is a flavivirus. Other closely related viruses cause similar diseases.
Transmission	Infection is transmitted by the bite of infected ticks. There is no direct person-to-person transmission. Some related viruses, also tick-borne, infect animals such as birds, deer (louping-ill), rodents and sheep.
Nature of the disease	Infection may induce an influenza-like illness, with a second phase of fever occurring in 10% of cases. Encephalitis develops during the second phase and may result in paralysis, permanent sequelae or death. Severity of illness increases with age.
Geographical distribution	Present in large parts of Europe, particularly Austria, the Baltic States (Estonia, Latvia, Lithuania), the Czech Republic, Hungary and the Russian Federation. The disease is seasonal, occurring mainly during the summer months in rural and forest areas at altitudes up to 1000 metres.
Risk for travellers	In endemic areas during the summer months, travellers are at risk when hiking or camping in rural or forest areas.
Prophylaxis	A vaccine against TBE is available (see Chapter 6).
Precautions	Avoid bites by ticks by wearing long trousers and closed footwear when hiking or camping in endemic areas. If a bite occurs, the tick should be removed as soon as possible.

TRYPANOSOMIASIS

1. *African trypanosomiasis* (sleeping sickness)

Cause	Protozoan parasites *Trypanosoma brucei gambiense* and *T. b. rhodesiense*.
Transmission	Infection occurs through the bite of infected tsetse flies. Humans are the main reservoir host for *T. b. gambiense*. Domestic cattle and wild animals, including antelopes, are the main animal reservoir of *T. b. rhodesiense*.

Nature of the disease	*T. b. gambiense* causes a chronic illness with onset of symptoms after a prolonged incubation period of weeks or months. *T. b. rhodesiense* causes a more acute illness, with onset a few days or weeks after the infected bite; often, there is a striking inoculation chancre. Initial clinical signs include severe headache, insomnia, enlarged lymph nodes, anaemia and rash. In the late stage of the disease, there is progressive loss of weight and involvement of the central nervous system. Without treatment, the disease is invariably fatal.
Geographical distribution	*T. b. gambiense* is present in foci in the tropical countries of western and central Africa. *T. b. rhodesiense* occurs in east Africa, extending south as far as Botswana.
Risk for travellers	Travellers are at risk in endemic regions if they visit rural areas for hunting, fishing, safari trips, sailing or other activities in remote areas.
Prophylaxis	None.
Precautions	Travellers should be aware of the risk in endemic areas and as far as possible avoid any contact with tsetse flies. However, bites are difficult to avoid because tsetse flies can bite through clothing. Travellers should be warned that tsetse flies bite during the day and are not repelled by available insect-repellent products. The bite is painful, which helps to identify its origin, and travellers should seek medical attention promptly if symptoms develop subsequently.

2. American trypanosomiasis (Chagas disease)

Cause	Protozoan parasite *Trypanosoma cruzi*.
Transmission	Infection is transmitted by blood-sucking triatomine bugs ("kissing bugs"). During feeding, infected bugs excrete trypanosomes, which can then contaminate the conjunctiva, mucous membranes, abrasions and skin wounds including the bite wound. Transmission also occurs by blood transfusion when blood has been obtained from an infected donor. Congenital infection is possible, due to parasites crossing the placenta during pregnancy. *T. cruzi* infects many species of wild and domestic animals as well as humans.
Nature of the disease	In adults, *T. cruzi* causes a chronic illness with progressive myocardial damage leading to cardiac arrhythmias and cardiac dilatation, and gastrointestinal involvement leading to mega-oesophagus and megacolon. *T. cruzi* causes acute illness in children, which is followed by chronic manifestations later in life.
Geographical distribution	American trypanosomiasis occurs in Mexico and in central and south America (as far south as central Argentina and Chile). The vector is found mainly in rural areas where it lives in the walls of poorly-constructed housing.
Risk for travellers	In endemic areas, travellers are at risk when trekking, camping or using poor-quality housing.
Precautions	Avoid exposure to blood-sucking bugs. Residual insecticides can be used to treat housing. Exposure can be reduced by the use of bednets in houses and camps.

TUBERCULOSIS

Cause	*Mycobacterium tuberculosis*, the tubercle bacillus. Humans can also become infected by bovine tuberculosis, caused by *M. bovis*.
Transmission	Infection is usually by direct airborne transmission from person to person.
Nature of the disease	Exposure to *Mycobacterium tuberculosis* may lead to infection, but most infections do not lead to disease. The risk of developing disease following infection is generally 5–10% during the lifetime, but may be increased by various factors, notably immunosuppression (e.g. advanced HIV infection).
	Multidrug resistance refers to strains of *M. tuberculosis* that are resistant to at least isoniazid and rifampicin. The resistant strains do not differ from other strains in infectiousness, likelihood of causing disease, or general clinical effects; however, if they do cause disease, treatment is more difficult and the risk of death will be higher.
Geographical distribution	Worldwide. The risk of infection differs between countries, as shown on the map of estimated TB incidence (page 83).
Risk for travellers	Low for most travellers. Long-term travellers (over 3 months) to a country with a higher incidence of tuberculosis than their own may have a risk of infection comparable to that for local residents. As well as the duration of the visit, living conditions are important in determining the risk of infection: high-risk settings include health facilities, shelters for the homeless, and prisons.
Prophylaxis	BCG vaccine is of limited use for travellers but may be advised for infants and young children in some situations (see Chapter 6).
Precautions	Travellers should avoid close contact with known tuberculosis patients. For travellers from low-incidence countries who may be exposed to infection in relatively high-incidence countries (e.g. health professionals, humanitarian relief workers, missionaries), a baseline tuberculin skin test is advisable in order to compare with retesting after return. If the skin reaction to tuberculin suggests recent infection, the traveller should receive, or be referred for, treatment for latent infection. Patients under treatment for tuberculosis should not travel until the treating physician has documented, by laboratory examination of sputum, that the patient is not infectious and therefore of no risk to others. The importance of completing the prescribed course of treatment should be stressed.

TYPHOID FEVER

Cause	*Salmonella typhi*, the typhus bacillus, which infects only humans. Similar paratyphoid and enteric fevers are caused by other species of *Salmonella*, which infect domestic animals as well as humans.
Transmission	Infection is transmitted by consumption of contaminated food or water. Occasionally direct faecal–oral transmission may occur. Shellfish taken from sewage-polluted beds are an important source of infection. Infection occurs through eating fruit and vegetables fertilized by night soil and eaten raw, and milk and milk products that have been contaminated by those in contact with them. Flies may transfer infection to foods, resulting in contamination

	that may be sufficient to cause human infection. Pollution of water sources may produce epidemics of typhoid fever, when large numbers of people use the same source of drinking-water.
Nature of the disease	A systemic disease of varying severity. Severe cases are characterized by gradual onset of fever, headache, malaise, anorexia and insomnia. Constipation is more common than diarrhoea in adults and older children. Without treatment, the disease progresses with sustained fever, bradycardia, hepatosplenomegaly, abdominal symptoms and, in some cases, pneumonia. In white-skinned patients, pink spots (papules), which fade on pressure, appear on the skin of the trunk in up to 50% of cases. In the third week, untreated cases develop additional gastrointestinal and other complications, which may prove fatal. Around 2–5% of those who contract typhoid fever become chronic carriers, as bacteria persist in the biliary tract after symptoms have resolved.
Geographical distribution	Worldwide. The disease occurs most commonly in association with poor standards of hygiene in food preparation and handling and where sanitary disposal of sewage is lacking.
Risk for travellers	Generally low risk for travellers, except in parts of north and west Africa, in south Asia and in Peru. Elsewhere, travellers are usually at risk only when exposed to low standards of hygiene with respect to food handling, control of drinking-water quality, and sewage disposal.
Prophylaxis	Vaccination (see Chapter 6).
Precautions	Observe all precautions against exposure to foodborne and waterborne infections (see Chapter 3).

TYPHUS FEVER (epidemic louse-borne typhus)

Cause	*Rickettsia prowazekii.*
Transmission	The disease is transmitted by the human body louse, which becomes infected by feeding on the blood of patients with acute typhus fever. Infected lice excrete rickettsia onto the skin while feeding on a second host, who becomes infected by rubbing louse faecal matter or crushed lice into the bite wound. There is no animal reservoir.
Nature of the disease	The onset is variable but often sudden, with headache, chills, high fever, prostration, coughing and severe muscular pain. After 5–6 days, a macular skin eruption (dark spots) develops first on the upper trunk and spreads to the rest of the body but usually not to the face, palms of the hands or soles of the feet. The case-fatality rate is up to 40% in the absence of specific treatment. Louse-borne typhus fever is the only rickettsial disease that can cause explosive epidemics.
Geographical distribution	Typhus fever occurs in colder (i.e. mountainous) regions of central and east Africa, central and south America and Asia. In recent years, most outbreaks have taken place in Burundi, Ethiopia and Rwanda. Typhus fever occurs in conditions of overcrowding and poor hygiene, such as prisons and refugee camps.

Risk for travellers	Very low for most travellers. Humanitarian relief workers may be exposed in refugee camps and other settings characterized by crowding and poor hygiene.
Prophylaxis	None.
Precautions	Cleanliness is important in preventing infestation by body lice. Insecticidal powders are available for body-louse control and treatment of clothing for those at high risk of exposure.

YELLOW FEVER

Cause	The yellow fever virus, an arbovirus of the *Flavivirus* genus.
Transmission	Yellow fever in urban and some rural areas is transmitted by the bite of infective *Aedes aegypti* mosquitoes and by other mosquitoes in the forests of south America. The mosquitoes bite during daylight hours. Transmission occurs at altitudes up to 2500 metres. Yellow fever virus infects humans and monkeys.
	In jungle and forest areas, monkeys are the main reservoir of infection, with transmission from monkey to monkey carried out by mosquitoes. The infective mosquitoes may bite humans who enter the forest area, usually causing sporadic cases or small outbreaks.
	In urban areas, monkeys are not involved and infection is transmitted among humans by mosquitoes. Introduction of infection into densely populated urban areas can lead to large epidemics of yellow fever.
	In Africa, an intermediate pattern of transmission is common in humid savannah regions. Mosquitoes infect both monkeys and humans, causing localized outbreaks.
Nature of the disease	Although some infections are asymptomatic, most lead to an acute illness characterized by two phases. Initially, there is fever, muscular pain, headache, chills, anorexia, nausea and/or vomiting, often with bradycardia. About 15% of patients progress to a second phase after a few days, with resurgence of fever, development of jaundice, abdominal pain, vomiting and haemorrhagic manifestations; half of these patients die 10–14 days after onset of illness.
Geographical distribution	The yellow fever virus is endemic in some tropical areas of Africa and central and south America (see map, page 84). The number of epidemics has increased since the early 1980s. Other countries are considered to be at risk of introduction of yellow fever due to the presence of the vector and suitable primate hosts (including Asia, where yellow fever has never been reported).
Risk for travellers	Travellers are at risk in all areas where yellow fever is endemic. The risk is greatest for visitors who enter forest and jungle areas.
Prophylaxis	Vaccination (see Chapter 6). In some countries, yellow fever vaccination is mandatory for visitors (see country list).
Precautions	Avoid mosquito bites during the day as well as at night (see Chapter 3).

Further reading

Disease outbreak news: http://www.who.int/disease-outbreak-news/index.html

Weekly epidemiological record: http://www.who.int/wer/

Chin J, ed. *Control of communicable diseases manual*, 17th ed. Washington, DC, American Public Health Association, 2000.

Cholera: basic facts for travellers: http://www.who.int/emc/diseases/cholera/factstravellers.html

WHO information on infectious diseases: http://www.who.int/emc/diseases/index.html; http://www.who.int/infectious-disease-news

Cholera, 2000–2001

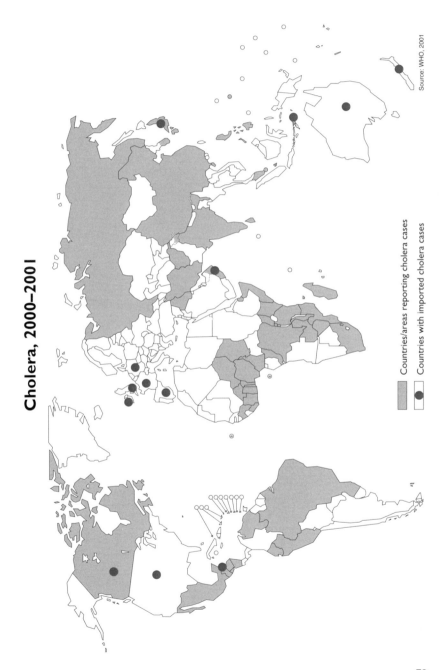

Source: WHO, 2001

Countries/areas reporting cholera cases

Countries with imported cholera cases

73

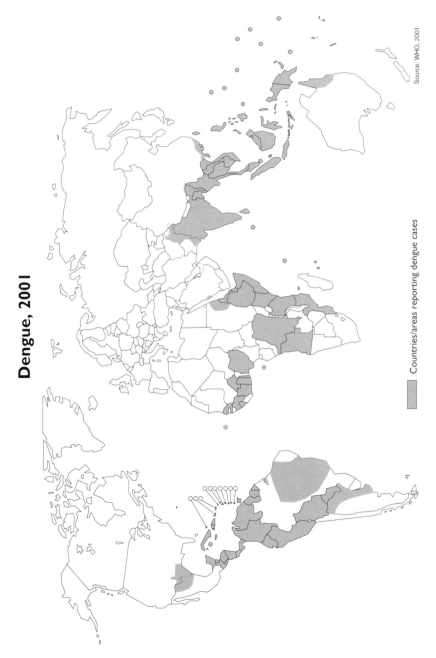

Dengue, 2001

Source: WHO, 2001

Countries/areas reporting dengue cases

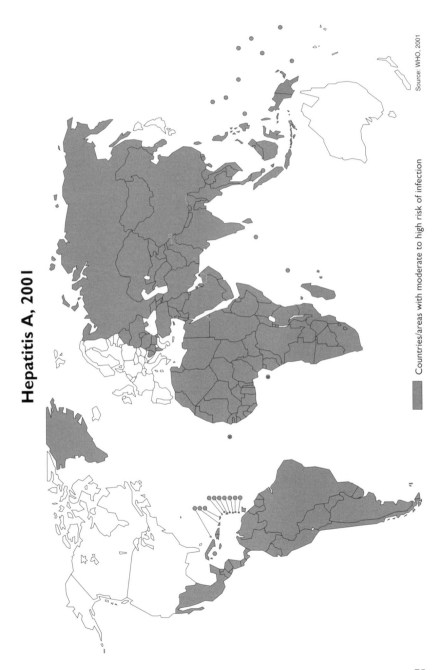

Hepatitis A, 2001

Countries/areas with moderate to high risk of infection

Source: WHO, 2001

Hepatitis B, 2001

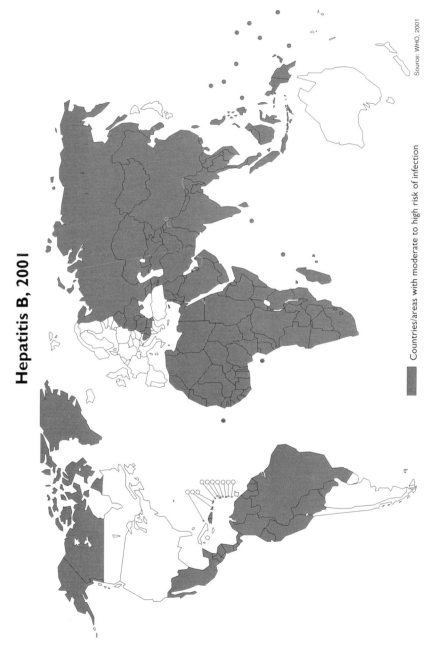

Source: WHO, 2001

Countries/areas with moderate to high risk of infection

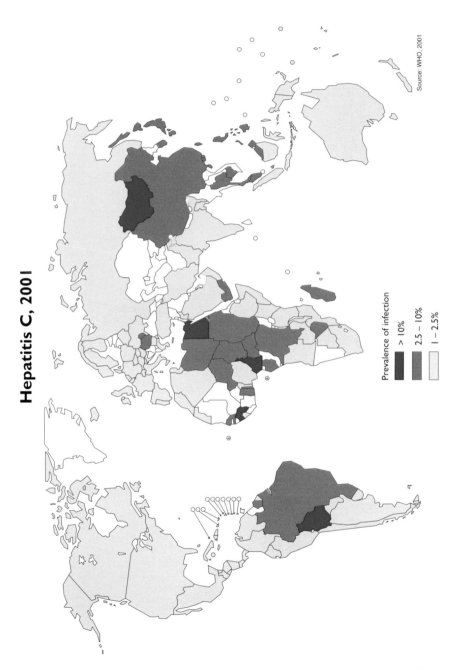

Hepatitis C, 2001

Source: WHO, 2001

Prevalence of infection

> 10%

2.5 – 10%

1 – 2.5%

HIV infection, end 1999

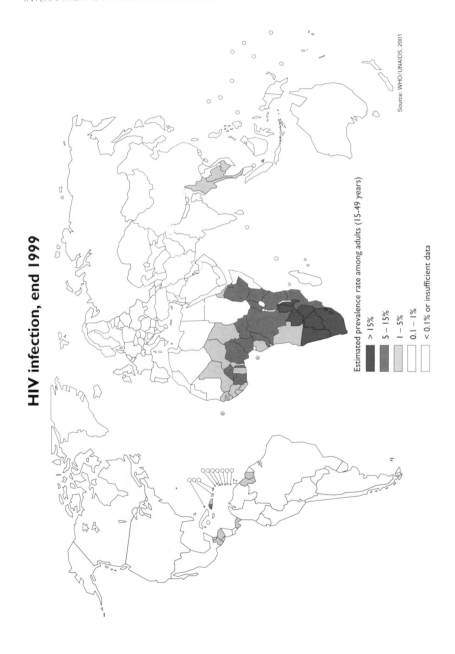

Source: WHO/UNAIDS, 2001

Estimated prevalence rate among adults (15-49 years)

- > 15%
- 5 – 15%
- 1 – 5%
- 0.1 – 1%
- < 0.1 % or insufficient data

Japanese encephalitis, 2001

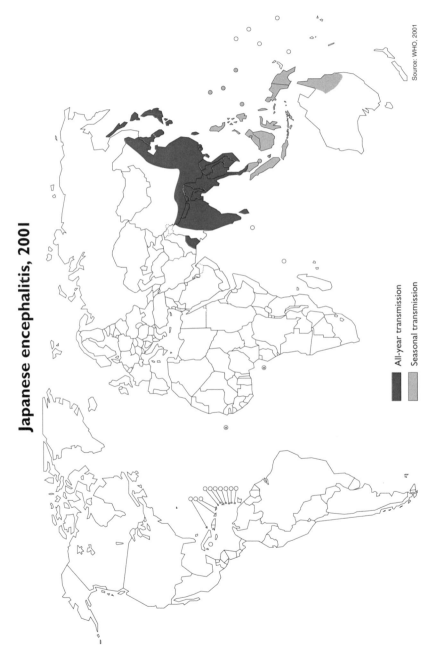

Source: WHO, 2001

All-year transmission
Seasonal transmission

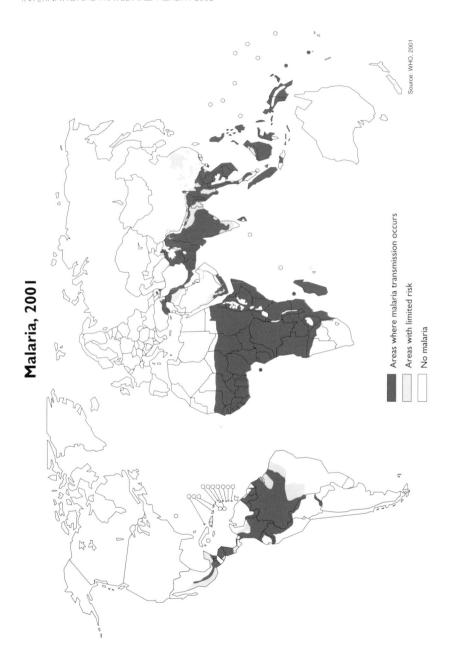

Malaria, 2001

Source: WHO, 2001

- Areas where malaria transmission occurs
- Areas with limited risk
- No malaria

Poliomyelitis, 2001

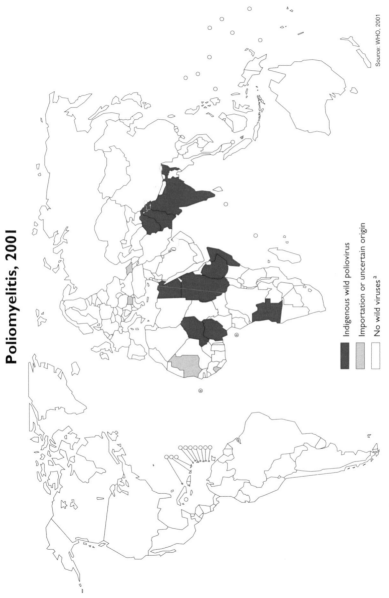

Source: WHO, 2001

■ Indigenous wild poliovirus

▨ Importation or uncertain origin

□ No wild viruses [a]

[a] Countries bordering on areas where wild poliovirus transmission occurs should be considered to pose a risk for travellers.
The Democratic Republic of the Congo should be considered as continuing to pose a risk, although no virus has been detected in that country for over a year.

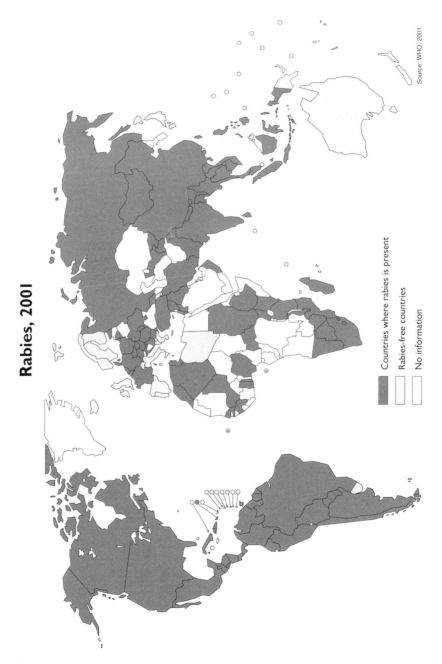

Rabies, 2001

Countries where rabies is present

Rabies-free countries

No information

Source: WHO, 2001

Tuberculosis, 2000

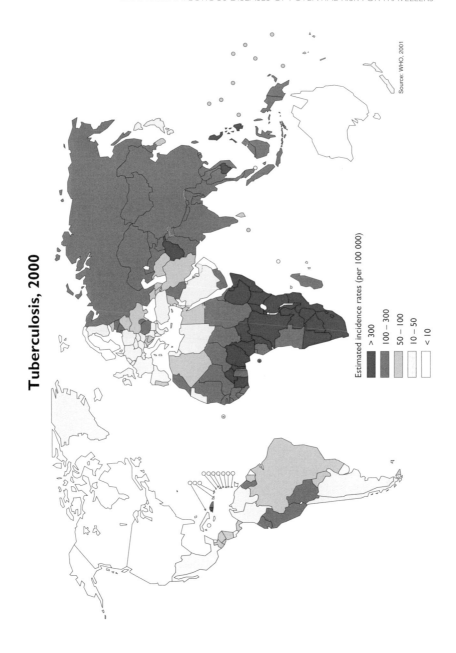

Source: WHO, 2001

Estimated incidence rates (per 100 000)

> 300
100 – 300
50 – 100
10 – 50
< 10

Yellow fever, 2001

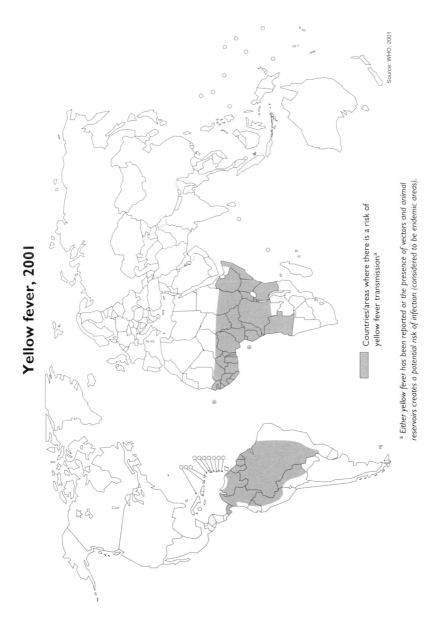

Source: WHO, 2001

Countries/areas where there is a risk of yellow fever transmission[a]

[a] *Either yellow fever has been reported or the presence of vectors and animal reservoirs creates a potential risk of infection (considered to be endemic areas).*

CHAPTER 6

Vaccine-preventable diseases, vaccines and vaccination

General considerations

Vaccination is the administration of a vaccine to stimulate a protective immune response that will prevent disease in the vaccinated person if contact with the corresponding infectious agent occurs subsequently. Thus vaccination, if successful, results in immunization: the vaccinated person has been immunized. In practice, the terms "vaccination" and "immunization" are often used interchangeably.

Disease prevention

Vaccination is a highly effective method of preventing certain infectious diseases. For the individual, and for society in terms of public health, prevention is better and more cost-effective than cure. Vaccines are generally very safe and adverse reactions are uncommon. Routine immunization programmes protect most of the world's children from a number of infectious diseases that previously claimed millions of lives each year. For travellers, vaccination offers the possibility of avoiding a number of dangerous infections that may be encountered abroad. However, vaccines have not yet been developed against several of the most life-threatening infections, including malaria and HIV/AIDS.

Vaccination and other precautions

Despite their success in preventing disease, vaccines do not fully protect 100% of the recipients. The vaccinated traveller should not assume that there is no risk of catching the disease(s) against which he/she has been vaccinated. All additional precautions against infection (see Chapter 5) should be followed carefully, regardless of any vaccines or other medication that have been administered. These same precautions are important in reducing the risk of acquiring diseases for which no vaccines exist.

Planning before travel

The protective effect of vaccines takes some time to develop following vaccination. The immune response of the vaccinated individual will become fully effective within a period of time that varies according to the vaccine, the number of doses required and whether the individual has previously been vaccinated against the same disease. For this reason, travellers are advised to consult a travel medicine clinic or personal physician 4–6 weeks before departure if the travel destination is one where exposure to any vaccine-preventable diseases may occur.

Vaccine schedules and administration

The vaccines that may be recommended or considered for travellers are shown in Table 6.1. The schedule for administration of each vaccine is given, together with other information for each of the vaccine-preventable diseases, on pages 89–127. Time intervals for administration of vaccines requiring more than one dose are recommended; some slight variation can be made to accommodate the needs of travellers who may not be able to complete the schedule exactly as recommended. In general, it is acceptable to lengthen the time intervals between doses, but significant shortening of the intervals is not recommended.

The route of administration differs for individual vaccines and is critical for induction of the protective immune response. For injectable vaccines, the route of injection — subcutaneous, intramuscular or intradermal — determines the gauge and length of the needle to be used.

Safe injections

The same high standard of injection safety should be applied to the administration of vaccines as to any other injection. A sterile needle and syringe should be used for each injection and disposed of safely.

WHO recommends the use of single-use ("auto-disable") syringes or disposable monodose preparations whenever possible. Syringes should not be recapped (to avoid needle-stick injuries) and should be disposed of in a way that is safe to the recipient, the provider and the community.

Multiple vaccines

All commonly used vaccines can be given simultaneously at separate sites at least 2 cm apart. However, certain vaccines commonly cause local reactions, which may be accentuated if a number of vaccines are given simultaneously. If possible, these vaccines should be given on separate occasions unless financial and time constraints dictate otherwise. Inactivated vaccines do not generally interfere with other inactivated or live vaccines and can be given simultaneously with, or at any time in relation to, other vaccines without prejudicing immune responses.

A number of combined vaccines are now available, providing protection against more than one disease, and new combinations are likely to become available in future years. For routine vaccination, the combined diphtheria/tetanus/pertussis (DTP) and measles/mumps/rubella (MMR) vaccines are in widespread use in children. Other examples of currently available combination vaccines are hepatitis A+B and hepatitis A + typhoid. In addition, other combination vaccines are available in certain countries: these include IPV+DTP, IPV+DTP+Hib and IPV+DTP+HepB+Hib.[1]

In adults, the combined diphtheria–tetanus vaccine (with reduced diphtheria—Td) is generally used in preference to monovalent (single-disease) vaccine.

Combined vaccines offer important advantages for travellers, by reducing the number of injections required and the amount of time involved, so aiding compliance. Combination vaccines are just as safe and effective as the individual single-disease vaccines.

Choice of vaccines for travel

Vaccines for travellers include: (1) those that are used routinely, particularly in children; (2) others that may be advised before travel; (3) those that, in some situations, are mandatory.

Most of the vaccines that are routinely administered in childhood require periodic booster doses throughout life to maintain an effective level of immunity. Adults in their country of residence often neglect to keep up the schedule of booster vaccinations, particularly if the risk of infection is low. Some older adults may never have been vaccinated at all. It is important to realize that diseases such as diphtheria and poliomyelitis, which no longer occur in most industrialized countries, may be present in those visited by travellers. Pretravel precautions should include booster doses of routine vaccines if the regular schedule has not been followed, or a full course of primary immunization for people who have never been vaccinated.

---

[1] IPV = inactivated poliomyelitis vaccine; Hib = *Haemophilus influenzae* type b [vaccine]; HepB = hepatitis B [vaccine].

Other vaccines will be advised on the basis of a travel risk assessment for the individual traveller (see also Chapter 1). In deciding which vaccines would be appropriate, the following factors are to be considered for each vaccine:

— risk of exposure to the disease
— age, health status, vaccination history
— special risk factors
— reactions to previous vaccine doses, allergies
— risk of infecting others
— cost.

Mandatory vaccination, as authorized by the International Health Regulations, nowadays concerns only yellow fever. Yellow fever vaccination is carried out for two different reasons: (1) to protect the *individual* in areas where there is a risk of yellow fever infection; and (2) to protect vulnerable *countries* from importation of the yellow fever virus. Travellers should therefore be vaccinated if they visit a country where there is a risk of exposure to yellow fever. They *must* be vaccinated if they visit a country that requires yellow fever vaccination

Table 6.1 **Vaccines for travellers**

Category	Vaccine
1. Routine vaccination	Diphtheria/tetanus/pertussis (DTP) Hepatitis B (HBV) *Haemophilus influenzae* type b (Hib) Measles (MMR) Poliomyelitis (OPV or IPV)[a]
2. Selective use for travellers	Cholera Influenza Hepatitis A (HAV) Japanese encephalitis Lyme disease Meningococcal meningitis Pneumococcal disease Rabies Tick-borne encephalitis Tuberculosis (BCG) Typhoid fever Yellow fever (for individual protection)
3. Mandatory vaccination	Yellow fever (for protection of vulnerable countries) Meningococcal meningitis (for Hajj, Umra)

[a] OPV = oral poliomyelitis vaccine; IPV = inactivated poliomyelitis vaccine.

as a condition of entry; this condition applies to all travellers who arrive from (including airport transit) a yellow fever endemic country.

Vaccination against meningococcal disease is required by Saudi Arabia for pilgrims visiting Mecca for the Hajj and is also required by some countries for returning pilgrims after the Hajj.

Travellers should be provided with a written record of all vaccines administered (patient-retained record), preferably using the international vaccination certificate (which is required in the case of yellow fever vaccination).

Vaccines for routine use

DIPHTHERIA

Disease

Diphtheria is a bacterial disease caused by *Corynebacterium diphtheriae*. The infection commonly affects the throat and may lead to obstruction of the airways and death. Transmission is from person to person, through close physical contact, and is increased in overcrowded and poor socioeconomic conditions. Exotoxin-induced damage occurs to organs such as the heart. Nasal diphtheria may be mild, and chronic carriage of the organism frequently occurs; asymptomatic infections are common. A cutaneous form of diphtheria is common in tropical countries and may be important in transmission of the infection.

Occurrence

Diphtheria is found worldwide, although it is not common in industrialized countries because of long-standing routine use of DTP vaccine. Recently, large epidemics have occurred in several east European countries.

Risk for travellers

Potentially life-threatening illness and severe, lifelong complications are possible in incompletely immunized individuals.

Vaccine

All travellers should be up to date with the vaccine, which is usually given as "triple vaccine"—DTP (diphtheria/tetanus/pertussis). After the initial course of three doses, additional doses may be given as DT until 7 years of age, after which a vaccine with reduced diphtheria content (Td) is given. Since both tetanus toxoid (see below) and diphtheria toxoid can reasonably be given on a booster basis about every 10 years, there is little reason to use monovalent diphtheria vaccine.

Precautions and contraindications

Avoid diphtheria-containing vaccines if a severe or life-threatening reaction has occurred to a previous dose. Use a vaccine with reduced diphtheria content (Td) from age 7 years onwards.

TETANUS

Disease

Tetanus is acquired through environmental exposure to the spores of *Clostridium tetani*, which are present in soil worldwide. The disease is caused by the action of a potent neurotoxin produced by the bacterium in dead tissue (e.g. dirty wounds). Clinical symptoms of tetanus are muscle spasms, initially muscles of mastication causing trismus or "lockjaw", which results in a characteristic facial expression—risus sardonicus. Trismus can be followed by sustained spasm of the back muscles (opisthotonus) and by spasms of other muscles. Finally, mild external stimuli may trigger generalized, tetanic seizures, which contribute to the serious complications of tetanus (dysphagia, aspiration pneumonia) and lead to death unless intense supportive treatment is rapidly initiated.

Occurrence

Dirty wounds can become infected with the tetanus spores anywhere in the world.

Risk for travellers

Every traveller should be fully protected against tetanus. Almost any form of injury, from a simple laceration to a motor-vehicle accident, can expose the individual to the spores.

Vaccine

All travellers should be up to date with the vaccine. The primary immunizing course of three doses of DTP is given in the first months of life. Booster doses are most easily given as Td, but certainly all doses given to individuals aged 7 years and above should be Td. A booster dose of Td should generally be used in preference to tetanus toxoid (TT) immediately following trauma. However, no such booster is needed if the last dose was given less than 5 (for dirty wounds) to 10 years (for clean wounds) previously.

Precautions and contraindications

Mild local reactions occur in up to 95% of vaccine recipients. Reactions increase in frequency and severity as the number of doses increases. After booster doses of TT, 50–80% of people experience some pain or tenderness at the injection site. True hypersensitivity reactions to TT occur very rarely.

PERTUSSIS

Disease

Pertussis (whooping cough) is a highly contagious acute bacterial disease involving the respiratory tract and caused by *Bordetella pertussis*. It is transmitted by direct contact with airborne discharges from the respiratory mucous membranes of infected persons. It causes a severe cough of several weeks' duration with a characteristic whoop, often with cyanosis and vomiting. In young infants, the cough may be absent and disease may manifest with spells of apnoea. Although pertussis can occur at any age, most serious cases and fatalities are observed in early infancy and mainly in developing countries. Major complications include pneumonia, encephalitis and malnutrition (due to repeated vomiting). Vaccination is the most rational approach to pertussis control.

Occurrence

Worldwide, *B. pertussis* causes at least 20 million cases of pertussis, 90% of which occur in developing countries, with an estimated 200 000 to 300 000 fatalities each year.

Risk for travellers

Unprotected infants are at high risk, but *all* children and young adults are at increased risk if they are not fully immunized. Exposure to pertussis is greater in developing countries, so children up to 7 years of age should be protected by vaccination. Pertussis vaccine is not generally recommended beyond 7 years.

Vaccine

All travellers should be up to date with the vaccine. Both whole-cell (wP) and acellular (aP) pertussis vaccines provide excellent protection. However, protection declines with time and probably extends only a few years. For several decades, wP vaccines have been widely used in national childhood vaccination programmes; aP vaccines, which cause fewer adverse effects, have been developed and are now being licensed in several countries. Both wP and aP are usually administered in combination with diphtheria and tetanus toxoids (DTwP or DTaP). Three doses are required for initial protection.

Precautions and contraindications

Pertussis-containing vaccines are not used after the seventh birthday. Whole-cell vaccines should not be given to children with an evolving neurological disease (e.g. uncontrolled epilepsy or progressive encephalopathy). Minor adverse effects such as local redness and swelling and fever are common after wP; prolonged crying and seizures are less common (<1 in 100) and hypotonic–hyporesponsive episodes are uncommon (<1 in 2000). Acellular vaccines cause significantly fewer reactions. The DTaP vaccines have proved to be significantly less reactogenic than the DTwP vaccines in terms of high fever, seizures and hypotonic–hyporesponsiveness episodes. The local reactogenicity of aP vaccines seems to increase with successive doses.

Type of vaccine:	Tetanus as toxoid; diphtheria as toxoid; pertussis as whole-cell or acellular preparation. May also be monovalent (TT), or bivalent (DT, Td)
Number of doses:	At least three, given i.m.
Schedule:	6, 10 and 14 weeks of age
Booster:	3–4 years of age; Td booster every 10 years
Contraindications:	Adverse reaction to a previous dose. Avoid wP vaccine in an evolving neurological disease (e.g. uncontrolled epilepsy, progressive encephalopathy)
Adverse reactions:	Mild local or systemic reaction is common
Before departure:	As long as possible. Some protection after second dose
Recommended for:	All, but particularly aid/health care workers
Special precautions:	Reduced diphtheria (Td instead of DT) content and no pertussis from 7 years of age

HAEMOPHILUS INFLUENZAE TYPE B

Disease

Haemophilus influenzae type b (Hib) is a common cause of bacterial meningitis and a number of other serious and potentially life-threatening conditions, including pneumonia, epiglottitis, osteomyelitis, septic arthritis and sepsis in infants and older children.

Occurrence

Hib is estimated to cause at least 3 million cases of serious disease and hundreds of thousands of deaths annually, worldwide. The most important manifestations of disease, namely pneumonia and meningitis, are seen mainly in children under 5 years of age, particularly in infants. Rarely occurring in infants under 3 months or after the age of 6 years, the disease burden is highest between 4 and 18 months of age. Hib is the dominant cause of sporadic (non-epidemic) bacterial meningitis in this age group, and is frequently associated with severe neurological sequelae despite prompt and adequate antibiotic treatment. In developing countries, it is estimated that 2–3 million cases of Hib pneumonia occur each year. The disease has practically disappeared in countries where routine vaccination of children is carried out.

Risk for travellers

All unprotected children are at risk at least up to the age of 5 years, and the risk may be increased by travel from a country with relatively low incidence to one where incidence is high.

Vaccine

All children who are not up to date with this vaccine should be offered it. Conjugate Hib vaccines have dramatically reduced the incidence of Hib meningitis in infants and of nasopharyngeal colonization by Hib. The vaccine is often given as a combined preparation with DTP or poliomyelitis vaccine. Hib vaccine is not yet used routinely in many developing countries where there is continuing high prevalence of the disease.

Precautions and contraindications

No serious side-effects have been recorded, and no contraindications are known, except for occasional hypersensitivity to a previous dose of the vaccine. All conjugate vaccines have an excellent safety record, and, where tested, do not interfere substantially with the immunogenicity of other vaccines given simultaneously.

Type of vaccine:	Conjugate
Number of doses:	Three or four depending on manufacturer and type of vaccine, given s.c.
Schedule:	6, 10 and 14 weeks of age

Contraindications:	Hypersensitivity to previous dose
Adverse reactions:	Mild local reaction
Before departure:	Full course up to date before departure
Recommended for:	All children up to 5 years of age
Special precautions:	None

HEPATITIS B

Disease and occurrence

See Chapter 5.

Risk for travellers

While only certain categories of traveller are clearly at risk because of their planned activities, any traveller may be involved in an accident or medical emergency that requires surgery. The vaccine should be considered for virtually all travellers to highly endemic areas. It can be administered to infants from birth. At particular risk are those who expose themselves to potentially infected blood or blood-derived fluids, or who have unprotected sexual contact. Principal risky activities include health care (medical, dental, laboratory or other) that entails direct exposure to human blood; receipt of a transfusion of blood that has not been tested for HBV; and dental, medical or other exposure to needles (e.g. acupuncture, piercing, tattooing or injecting drug use) that have not been appropriately sterilized. In addition, in less developed countries, skin lesions in children or adults suffering from impetigo, scabies or scratched insect bites may play a role in disease transmission if there is direct exposure to open wounds.

Vaccine

Hepatitis B vaccine produced both from plasma and by recombinant DNA technology (usually in yeast) is available; the two types are equally safe and effective. Three doses of vaccine constitute the complete series; the first two doses are usually given 1 month apart, with the third dose 1–12 months later. In some countries, a two-dose schedule has been introduced for adolescents, with the second dose given 6–12 months after the first. Immunization provides protection for at least 15 years. Because of the prolonged incubation period of hepatitis B, some protection will be afforded to most travellers following the second dose given before travel, provided that the final dose is given upon return. If the trip is to be a long one, a schedule of rapid vaccination is preferred (see below). Prevaccination screening to determine immune status is generally not cost-effective in people from industrialized countries, but may be helpful in those from developing countries who have a high probability of having had asymptomatic infection during childhood.

The standard schedule of administration is three doses, given as follows: day 0; 1 month; 6–12 months.

A rapid schedule of administration of monovalent hepatitis B vaccine may be considered as follows: day 0; 1 month; 2 months.

In some countries of the European Union, another rapid schedule has been licensed, with doses given as follows: : day 0; day 7; day 21.

However, if either of the two rapid schedules is used, it is recommended that an additional dose is given after 6–12 months.

A combination vaccine that provides protection against both hepatitis A and hepatitis B may be considered for travellers potentially exposed to both organisms. This inactivated vaccine is administered as follows: day 0; 1 month; 6 months.

Precautions and contraindications

Hepatitis B vaccines are extremely safe. Mild, transient local reactions occur commonly, but anaphylactic reactions are extremely rare. Despite extensive press coverage of the subject, no scientific evidence exists to support the suggestion that hepatitis B vaccine might be a cause of multiple sclerosis.

Type of vaccine:	Inactivated
Number of doses:	Three (volume varies with manufacturer), given i.m. in the deltoid muscle; for some products, only two doses for adolescents
Schedule:	Several options (see text above)
Contraindications:	Adverse reaction to previous dose
Adverse reactions:	Local soreness and redness
Before departure:	Second dose at least 2 weeks before departure
Recommended for:	All who are not up to date
Special precautions:	Particularly important for travellers from low-incidence areas to hyperendemic regions and for those at high risk

MEASLES

Disease

Measles is a highly contagious infection; before vaccines became available this disease had affected most people by the time of adolescence. In developing countries, it still causes up to 875 000 deaths annually. The disease typically presents with fever, red rash and runny nose. Common complications include middle-ear infection and pneumonia. Transmission is primarily by large respiratory droplets. Measles is found worldwide, and occurs in a seasonal pattern. Transmission increases during the late winter and early spring in temperate climates, and after the rainy season in tropical climates. Epidemics occur every 2 or 3 years in areas where there is low vaccine coverage. In countries where measles has been largely eliminated, cases imported from other countries remain an important continuing source of infection.

Occurrence

Measles occurs worldwide, although far fewer cases now occur in industrialized countries and indigenous transmission has virtually stopped in the Americas. Virus transmission still occurs in most tropical countries.

Risk for travellers

Travellers who are not fully immunized against measles are at risk when visiting developing countries.

Vaccine

All travellers from 6 months of age who have not been immunized should be offered measles vaccine. One dose of vaccine in infancy protects around 80–90% of recipients for more than 20 years. The measles/mumps/rubella triple (MMR) or measles/rubella (MR) vaccine is given in many countries instead of monovalent measles vaccine. The appropriate age for administration is either 9 months or 12–15 months, depending on epidemiological and other factors relating to all three diseases. Many countries give additional doses either at a particular age (e.g. 5 years) or during mass campaigns.

Special attention must be paid to all children who have not been vaccinated against measles at the appropriate time. Measles is still common in many countries and travel in densely populated areas may favour transmission. For infants travelling to countries where measles is endemic, a dose of vaccine may be given as early as 6 months of age. However, children who receive the first dose between 6 and

8 months should also receive the scheduled dose at 9 months or 12–15 months of age.

It is generally recommended that individuals with a moderate degree of immune deficiency receive the vaccine if there is even a low risk of contracting measles infection from the community. There is a low level of risk in using measles vaccine in immunocompromised HIV-infected individuals. Where the risk of contracting measles infection is negligible, physicians who are able to monitor immune status, for instance CD4 counts, may prefer to avoid the use of measles vaccine.

Precautions and contraindications

Measles vaccine is generally extremely safe. However, since it is a live viral vaccine, it should be avoided during pregnancy. It should also be avoided if there is a known allergy to neomycin or gelatin, or if a severe reaction has occurred following a previous dose of measles (or MR or MMR) vaccine. Very rarely, encephalitis may follow measles vaccination. Measles vaccine is equally safe and effective when administered as a single vaccine or in combination. The mumps component may account for transient parotitis and, rarely, central nervous system symptoms due to aseptic meningitis. The rubella component may account for transient lymphadenopathy and, in 25% of rubella-susceptible women, joint symptoms.

Type of vaccine:	Live viral
Number of doses:	One, given i.m. or s.c., although many countries schedule more than one dose for high levels of control
Contraindications:	Pregnancy; adverse reaction to previous dose
Adverse reactions:	Malaise, fever, rash 5–12 days after vaccination, rarely encephalopathy
Before departure:	4 weeks
Recommended for:	All infants from 9 months of age,[1] children, young adults who have not had at least one dose previously, and adults who have no documented evidence of previous vaccination
Special precautions:	None

---

[1] Infants travelling to high-risk countries may have an additional dose as early as 6 months of age, as well as the scheduled dose at 9 or 12–15 months of age.

POLIOMYELITIS

Disease

Poliomyelitis is a disease of the central nervous system caused by three closely related enteroviruses, poliovirus types 1, 2 and 3. The virus is spread predominantly by the faecal–oral route, although rare outbreaks caused by contaminated food or water have occurred. After the virus enters the mouth, the primary site of infection is the intestine, although the virus can also be found in the pharynx. Poliomyelitis is also known as "infantile paralysis" because it most frequently causes paralysis in infants and young children: 60–70% of cases occur in children under 3 years of age and 90% in children under 5 years of age. The resulting paralysis is permanent, although some recovery of function is possible with physiotherapy. There is no cure.

Occurrence

Wild poliovirus transmission has ceased in almost all industrialized countries and much of the developing world (see map page 81). Remaining countries are expected to be free of poliomyelitis by 2005.

Risk for travellers

Until the disease has been certified as eradicated, the risk of acquiring it remains and travellers to endemic countries should be fully protected by vaccination. The consequences of infection are life-threatening or crippling. Infection and paralysis may occur in non-immune individuals and are by no means confined to infants. Infected travellers are potent vectors for transmission and possible reintroduction of the virus into polio-free zones now that worldwide eradication is near.

Vaccine

All travellers should be up to date with vaccination against poliomyelitis. There are two types of vaccine: inactivated (IPV), which is given by injection, and oral (OPV). OPV is composed of the three types of live attenuated polioviruses. Because of the low cost and ease of administration of the vaccine and its superiority in conferring intestinal immunity, OPV has been the vaccine of choice for controlling epidemic poliomyelitis in many countries. The immunity produced by OPV is apparently lifelong.

IPV is used in several European countries and the USA, either as the sole vaccine against poliomyelitis or in schedules combined with OPV. Although IPV suppresses pharyngeal excretion of wild poliovirus, this vaccine has only limited effects in reducing intestinal excretion of poliovirus. For unvaccinated older children and adults, the second dose is given 1–2 months after the first, and the third 6–12 months after the second. A booster dose is recommended after 4–6 years. IPV is also the vaccine of choice for travellers with no history of OPV use, as well as for immunocompromised individuals and their contacts and family members.

For those who have received three or more doses of OPV in the past, it is advisable to offer another dose of polio vaccine as a once-only dose to those travelling to endemic areas of the world. Any unimmunized individuals intending to travel to such an area require a complete course of vaccine. Countries differ in recommending IPV or OPV in these circumstances: IPV has the advantage of avoiding any risk of vaccine-associated paralytic poliomyelitis (VAPP), but is more expensive and may not stop faecal excretion of the virus.

Precautions and contraindications

Both IPV and OPV are very safe vaccines. Reactions to IPV are extremely rare and tend to be limited to allergic responses among persons already sensitive to either the formaldehyde or the antibiotics used in the preparation of the vaccine.

The major adverse event associated with OPV is VAPP. The risk of VAPP is higher after the first dose of OPV than after subsequent doses, ranging from 1 case per 1.4 million to 1 case per 3.4 million first doses administered. VAPP is more common in individuals who are immunocompromised, for whom IPV is the vaccine of choice.

Type of vaccine:	Live oral (OPV) or killed inactivated injectable (IPV)
Number of doses:	Four of OPV; three of IPV
Schedule:	OPV at 6, 10 and 14 weeks of age (plus a dose at birth in endemic countries). IPV at 2, 4 and 12–18 months
Booster:	One lifetime dose before travel to endemic countries
Contraindications:	None
Adverse reactions:	Very rarely VAPP following OPV
Before departure:	4 weeks
Recommended for:	All travellers to developing countries where poliomyelitis is still transmitted
Special precautions:	Immunocompromised travellers should receive IPV rather than OPV

Vaccines for selective use

Vaccines in this section need be offered only to travellers who are going to certain specified destinations. The decision to recommend a vaccine will depend on a travel risk assessment for the individual.

CHOLERA

Disease and occurrence

See Chapter 5.

Risk for travellers

Travellers are not at significant risk from cholera provided that simple precautions are taken to avoid potentially contaminated food and water. Currently available new vaccines are not necessary for most travellers: the sensible selection of clean drinking-water and food is more important than vaccination in preventing cholera, and even the vaccinated traveller should continue to be prudent about food and drink. Vaccination is advisable for those at increased risk of the disease, particularly emergency relief and health workers in refugee situations.

Vaccine

Cholera vaccine is not required as a condition of entry to any country. The two new cholera vaccines (live and killed), given orally, are safe and effective. They have been licensed and are commercially available in a limited number of countries, making possible their use as an option for travellers to high-risk situations in endemic areas. The killed vaccine confers high-grade (85–90%) protection for 6 months after the second dose. Protection remains as high as 62% after 3 years in vaccine recipients over 5 years of age. Killed cholera vaccine confers some level of cross-protection against *Escherichia coli* and therefore against "travellers' diarrhoea".

The traditional injectable cholera vaccine conveys incomplete, unreliable protection of short duration; it is not recommended.

Precautions and contraindications

Antibiotics and malaria prophylaxis with proguanil should both be avoided from 1 week before until 1 week after administration of the live oral attenuated vaccine. Vaccination should be completed at least 3 days before the first prophylactic dose of mefloquine (see page 143).

Type of vaccine:	Killed and live attenuated oral
Number of doses:	Two, one week apart (killed vaccine); one (live vaccine)
Contraindications:	Hypersensitivity to previous dose
Adverse reactions:	Mild local reaction of short duration; mild systemic reaction
Before to departure:	3 weeks (killed vaccine), 1 week (live vaccine)
Consider for:	Travellers to endemic areas
Special precautions:	No antibiotics from 1 week before until 1 week after vaccination (live vaccine). Avoid proguanil from 1 week before to 1 week after vaccination (live vaccine). Strict precautions regarding food, water and hygiene

HEPATITIS A

Disease and occurrence

Although hepatitis A is rarely fatal in children and young adults, most infected adults and some older children become ill and are unable to work for several weeks or months. The case-fatality rate exceeds 2% among those over 40 years of age and may be 4% for those aged 60 years or more. (See also Chapter 5.)

Risk for travellers

Hepatitis A is the most common vaccine-preventable infection of travellers. Travellers from industrialized countries are likely to be susceptible to infection and should receive the hepatitis A vaccine before travelling to developing countries. While people travelling to rural areas of developing countries are at particularly high risk of infection, in practice most cases occur among travellers staying in resorts and good-quality hotels. People born and raised in developing countries, and those born before 1945 in industrialized countries, have often been infected in childhood and are likely to be immune. For such individuals, it may be cost-effective to test for anti-HAV antibodies so that unnecessary vaccination can be avoided.

Vaccine

The vaccine should be considered for all travellers to highly endemic zones, and those at high risk of acquiring the disease should be strongly encouraged to accept vaccination. A safe and highly effective inactivated (killed) hepatitis A vaccine became available in 1992. Since antibodies induced by the vaccine are not detectable until 2 weeks after administration, travellers should be vaccinated 4 weeks before departure if possible. A booster dose given 6–24 months later is recommended. This schedule is expected to provide at least 10 years' protection.

In the case of emergency travel to a high-risk area, a dose of immunoglobulin (0.02 ml/kg), where this product is still available, may be given with the first dose of vaccine.

A combination hepatitis A/typhoid vaccine is available for those exposed to waterborne diseases. The vaccine is administered as a single dose, a minimum of 4 weeks before departure, and confers high levels of protection against both diseases. A second dose of hepatitis A vaccine is needed 6–12 months later and boosters of typhoid vaccine should be given at 3-yearly intervals.

Precautions and contraindications

Minor local and systemic reactions are fairly common.

Type of vaccine:	Inactivated, given i.m.
Number of doses:	Two
Schedule:	Second dose 6–24 months after the first
Booster:	May not be necessary—manufacturers propose at 10 years
Contraindications:	Hypersensitivity to previous dose
Adverse reactions:	Mild local reaction of short duration, mild systemic reaction
Before departure:	Protection 4 weeks after first dose; some protection immediately after first dose
Recommended for:	All non-immune travellers to highly endemic areas
Special precautions:	None

INFLUENZA

Disease and occurrence

See Chapter 5.

Risk for travellers

All travellers to areas of the world experiencing a seasonal (winter and spring) influenza outbreak are at potential risk of contracting the disease. Tourists are at risk because they often travel in crowded vehicles and visit crowded places—both situations that promote transmission. Elderly people, individuals with respiratory and cardiac disease, diabetes mellitus, or any immunosuppressive condition, and health care workers are particularly at risk. The impact of an attack of influenza during travel can range from highly inconvenient to life-threatening.

Vaccine

Influenza viruses constantly evolve, with rapid changes in their antigenic characteristics. To be effective, influenza vaccines need to stimulate immunity to the principal strains of virus circulating at the time. The vaccine contains three strains, with the composition being modified every year to ensure protection against the strains prevailing in each influenza season. Since the antigenic changes in circulating influenza viruses occur very rapidly, there may be significant differences between prevailing strains during the influenza seasons of the northern and southern hemispheres, which occur at different times of the year (November–March in the north and April–September in the south). The vaccine composition is adjusted for the hemisphere in which it will be used. Consequently, vaccine obtainable in one hemisphere may offer only partial protection against influenza infection in the other.

Travellers in the high-risk groups for influenza should be regularly vaccinated each year. Anyone travelling from one hemisphere to the other shortly before, or early during, the influenza season, should arrange vaccination as soon as possible after arriving at the travel destination. Vaccine for the opposite hemisphere is unlikely to be obtainable before arrival.

Precautions and contraindications

Mild local and/or systemic reactions are common. Vaccination is contraindicated in case of egg allergy.

Type of vaccine:	Inactivated non-infectious viral
Number of doses:	One, given s.c. or i.m.
Booster:	Annual; immunocompromised individuals should receive a second dose 4 weeks after the first
Contraindications:	Hypersensitivity to previous dose or severe hypersensitivity to egg
Adverse reactions:	Local pain and tenderness at injection site (20%), fever, malaise

Before departure:	2 weeks
Recommended for:	High-risk groups before the influenza season, and optional for travellers to countries currently in influenza season
Special precautions:	None

JAPANESE ENCEPHALITIS

Disease and occurrence

See Chapter 5.

Risk for travellers

The risk of infection with Japanese encephalitis (JE) for travellers to south-east Asia is low but varies with the season (being higher during the monsoon), the type of accommodation and the duration of exposure. Short stays in good hotels with limited likelihood of mosquito bites result in very low levels of risk. In contrast, campers in rural areas may be at high risk. No more than one case per year is diagnosed in civilian travellers worldwide.

Vaccine

The vaccine should be considered for all travellers to rural endemic zones if they intend to stay there for at least 2 weeks. Those at high risk should be strongly encouraged to accept vaccination. Three types of JE vaccine are currently in large-scale production and use: inactivated mouse-brain-derived vaccine (IMB), cell-culture-derived inactivated vaccine and cell-culture-derived live attenuated vaccine. Only the IMB vaccine is widely commercially available.

Precautions and contraindications

A hypersensitivity reaction to a previous dose is a contraindication. The vaccine should be avoided in pregnancy unless the likely risk favours its administration. Rare, but serious, neurological side-effects attributed to IMB vaccine have been reported from endemic as well as non-endemic regions. Allergic reactions to components of the vaccine occur occasionally. As such reactions may occur within 2 weeks of administration, it is advisable to ensure that the complete course of vaccine is administered well in advance of departure.

Type of vaccine:	Inactivated mouse-brain-derived
Number of doses:	Standard 3-dose schedule or reduced 2-dose schedule, s.c.
Schedule:	3 doses at days 0, 7 and 28; or 2 doses given 1–4 weeks apart (1.0 ml for adults, 0.5 ml for children)
Booster:	After 1 year and then 3-yearly
Contraindications:	Hypersensitivity to previous dose or to the vaccine preservative thiomersal
Adverse reactions:	Occasional mild local or systemic reaction; occasional severe reaction with generalized urticaria, hypotension and collapse
Before departure:	At least two doses before departure
Recommended for:	Travellers over 1 year of age and staying in endemic rural areas for more than 2 weeks
Special precautions:	Avoiding mosquito bites is as important as being immunized

LYME DISEASE

Disease and occurrence

See Chapter 5.

Risk for travellers

Travellers at risk include hikers and campers in forested areas of known infested regions during the tick season (spring to early aumtumn). They may be offered the vaccine as well as being advised to minimize exposure to ticks by using insect repellent and wearing clothes that cover as much skin area as possible.

Vaccine

Vaccine is available only in the USA and is strain-specific for that region. The vaccine is administered intramuscularly in three doses of 0.5 ml at day 0, 1 month and 12 months. The level of seroprotection is 76% after three doses but only 49% after two doses, clearly indicating that use of the vaccine should be supplemented by the other methods of personal protection. The vaccine is licensed for use in those aged 15–70 years and is well tolerated. At present, it is uncertain whether this vaccine will provide protection against infection with other strains of *B. burgdorferi*. Available data indicate that a booster dose of vaccine will probably be necessary a year after completion of the primary course.

Precautions and contraindications

Only mild reactions are reported after vaccination. Daily checks should be made for ticks, which should be removed at once. If erythema migrans (an expanding annular zone of reddening of the skin) is observed, medical guidance should be sought immediately. Soreness, redness and swelling at the injection site occur occasionally.

Type of vaccine:	Killed, specific for north America
Number of doses:	Three, at day 0, 1 month and 12 months
Booster:	Probably needed after 1 year
Contraindications:	Children under 15 years of age; adverse reaction to previous dose
Adverse reactions:	Local side-effects only
Before departure:	2 months
Recommended for:	Walkers, campers, etc. in infested countryside
Special precautions:	Check daily for ticks and erythema migrans

MENINGOCOCCAL MENINGITIS

Disease and occurrence

See Chapter 5.

Risk for travellers

Vaccination should be considered for travellers to countries where outbreaks of meningococcal meningitis are known to occur.

- Travellers to industrialized countries are exposed to the possibility of sporadic cases. Outbreaks of meningococcal C disease occur in schools, colleges, military barracks and other places where large numbers of adolescents and young adults congregate.

- Travellers to the sub-Saharan meningitis belt may be exposed to outbreaks of serogroup A disease with comparatively very high incidence rates. Long-term travellers living in close contact with the indigenous population may be at greater risk of infection.

- Pilgrims to Mecca are at risk. The quadrivalent vaccine, (A, C, Y, W-135) is currently required for visiting pilgrims.

Vaccine

The vaccine should be offered only to travellers at significant risk of infection (see above). Internationally licensed meningococcal vaccines are monovalent (group A or C), bivalent (groups A and C) or quadrivalent (groups A, C, Y, and W-135). The vaccines are purified, heat-stable, lyophilized capsular polysaccharides from meningococci of the respective serogroups. The recommended single dose of the reconstituted vaccine contains 50 µg of each of the individual polysaccharides.

Both group A and group C vaccines have documented short-term efficacy levels of 85–100% in older children and adults. However, group C vaccines do not prevent disease in children under 2 years of age, and the efficacy of group A vaccine in children under 1 year of age is unclear. Group Y and W-135 polysaccharides have been shown to be immunogenic only in children over 2 years of age.

A monovalent serogroup C conjugate vaccine has recently been licensed for use in children and adolescents. This conjugate (T-cell dependent) vaccine has enhanced immunogenicity, particularly for children under 2 years of age.

A protective antibody response occurs within 10–14 days of vaccination. In schoolchildren and adults, both group A and group C vaccines appear to provide protection for at least 3 years, but in children under 4 years, the levels of specific antibodies decline rapidly after 2–3 years.

The currently available group A and group C meningococcal vaccines are recommended for immunization of specific risk groups as well as for large-scale immunization, as appropriate, in connection with epidemic outbreaks of group A or C meningococcal disease. The group A and group C vaccines do not provide any protection against group B meningococci, which are the leading cause of endemic meningococcal disease in some countries.

Precautions and contraindications

These vaccines are very safe, and significant systemic reactions have been extremely rare. The most common adverse reactions are erythema and slight pain at the site of injection for 1–2 days. Fever exceeding 38.5 °C occurs in up to 2% of vaccinees. No significant change in safety or reactogenicity has been observed when the different group-specific polysaccharides are combined into bivalent or tetravalent meningococcal vaccines. Cross-protection does not occur and travellers already immunized with conjugate vaccine against serogroup C are not protected against other serogroups.

Those at high risk of type C infection may be vaccinated with the conjugate C vaccine, followed 2 weeks later by the polysaccharide vaccine. All other antigens may be administered simultaneously with the conjugate C vaccine. In the case of other conjugate vaccines containing either diphtheria or tetanus toxoid as the carrier protein, it is advisable to administer at a 1-month interval to avoid enhanced reactogenicity.

Type of vaccine:	Purified bacterial capsular polysaccharide
Number of doses:	One
Booster:	Every 3 years; protection lasts at least 2 years after infancy
Contraindications:	Serious adverse reaction to previous dose
Adverse reactions:	Occasional mild local reactions; rarely, slight fever
Before departure:	2 weeks
Consider for:	All travellers to countries in the sub-Saharan meningitis belt, students at risk from endemic disease; Hajj pilgrims (mandatory)
Special precautions:	Children under 2 years of age are not protected by the vaccine

PNEUMOCOCCAL DISEASE

Disease

The term "pneumococcal disease" refers to a group of clinical conditions caused by the bacterium *Streptococcus pneumoniae*. Invasive pneumococcal infections include pneumonia, meningitis and febrile bacteraemia; the common non-invasive conditions include otitis media, sinusitis and bronchitis. Infection is acquired by direct person-to-person contact via respiratory droplets or oral contact. There are many healthy, asymptomatic carriers of the bacteria. There is no animal reservoir or insect vector.

Several chronic conditions predispose to serious pneumococcal disease (see below). Increasing pneumococcal resistance to antibiotics underlines the importance of vaccination.

Occurrence

Pneumococcal diseases are a worldwide public health problem. *S. pneumoniae* is the leading cause of severe pneumonia in children under 5 years of age, causing over 1 million deaths each year, mainly in developing countries. In industrialized countries, most pneumococcal disease occurs in the elderly.

Risk for travellers

Travellers with certain chronic conditions are at increased risk of pneumococcal disease and should be vaccinated. These predisposing conditions include sickle-cell disease, other haemoglobinopathies, chronic renal failure, chronic liver disease, immunosuppression after organ transplantation and other etiological factors, asplenia and dysfunctional spleen, leaks of cerebrospinal fluid, diabetes mellitus and HIV infection.

Vaccine

The current polysaccharide vaccines contain capsular antigens of 23 serotypes, which cause 90% of pneumococcal infections. The vaccines are immunogenic in those over 2 years of age. Children under 2 years of age and immunocompromised individuals do not respond well to the vaccine. Vaccination provides a relative protection against pneumococcal pneumonia in healthy elderly individuals.

Pneumococcal vaccine is recommended for selected groups, above the age of 2 years, with increased risk of pneumococcal disease. In some countries, such as the USA, routine vaccination is recommended for everyone aged above 65 years.

A new generation of conjugate pneumococcal vaccines is now being evaluated. These vaccines contain 9–11 selected polysaccharides bound to a protein carrier, and induce a T-cell-dependent immune response. Conjugate vaccines are likely to be protective even in children below 2 years of age.

Precautions and contraindications

Pneumococcal polysaccharide vaccine is generally considered very safe. Mild, local reactions persisting for up to 48 hours are common; more severe local reactions are unusual. Moderate systemic reactions (e.g. fever and myalgia) are unusual and severe adverse effects (e.g. anaphylactic reactions) are rare.

Revaccination after 3–6 years may be considered for those in certain high-risk groups in whom immunity following vaccination is known to decline rapidly.

Type of vaccine:	Polysaccharide
Number of doses:	One, given s.c. or i.m.
Booster:	Can be considered after 5 years
Contraindications:	Adverse reaction to previous dose
Adverse reactions:	Mild local reactions
Before departure:	2 weeks
Recommended for:	Those at high risk (see text above)
Special precautions:	None

RABIES

Disease and occurrence

See Chapter 5.

Risk for travellers

The risk to travellers in endemic areas is proportional to their contact with potentially rabid animals. For instance, it is estimated that 13% of visitors to one country in south-east Asia come into contact with local animals. Veterinary workers and people who work in the streets of big-city slums where dogs roam wild are at the greatest risk. Most travellers in tourist resorts are at very low risk. There is a greater risk for children, however, who may have more contact with animals and may not report suspect incidents. It is prudent to avoid walking in populated areas where dogs roam. Following suspect contact, especially bites or scratches, medical advice should be sought at once at a competent medical centre, ideally in the capital city. First-aid measures should be started immediately (see also Chapter 5).

Vaccine

Vaccination against rabies is carried out in two distinct situations:

— to protect those who are likely to be exposed to rabies, i.e. pre-exposure vaccination;
— to prevent the establishment of rabies infection after exposure has taken place, usually following the bite of an animal suspected of having rabies, i.e. post-exposure vaccination.

The vaccines used for pre-exposure and post-exposure vaccination are the same, but the schedule of administration differs according to the type of application. Modern vaccines of cell-culture origin are safer and more effective than the older vaccines, which were produced in brain tissue, and are now used in most countries.

Pre-exposure immunization should be offered to people at high risk of exposure, such as laboratory staff working with rabies virus, veterinarians, animal handlers and wildlife officers, and to other individuals living or travelling in areas where rabies is endemic. Pre-exposure immunization is advisable for children in endemic areas, where they provide an easy target for rabid animals.

Such immunization should preferably consist of three full intramuscular doses of cell-culture rabies vaccine given on days 0, 7 and 21–28 (a few days' variation in the timing is not important). For adults, the vaccine should always be administered in the deltoid area of the arm; for young children, the anterolateral area of the thigh is also acceptable. The gluteal area should never be used, since vaccine administration in this area results in lower neutralizing antibody titres.

Where feasible, and particularly in individuals at occupational risk, the presence of virus-neutralizing antibodies should be confirmed using serum samples collected 1–3 weeks after the final dose.

Tissue-culture or purified duck-embryo rabies vaccines of potency at least 2.5 IU/dose induce adequate antibody titres when carefully administered intradermally in 0.1 ml volumes on days 0, 7 and 28. Vaccination by the intradermal route is less immunogenic than intramuscular vaccination, but offers cost savings since the dose is only 0.1 ml per intradermal site.

For post-exposure vaccination see Chapter 5.

Precautions and contraindications

Modern rabies vaccines are well tolerated. The frequency of minor adverse reactions (local pain, erythema, swelling and pruritus) varies widely from one report to another. Occasional systemic reactions (malaise, generalized aches and headaches) have been noted after both intramuscular and intradermal injections.

Type of vaccine:	Modern vaccine (cell-cultured or embryonated egg vaccine)
Number of doses:	Three, on days 0, 7 and 21–28, given i.m. (1 ml/dose) or i.d. (0.1 ml/dose)
Booster:	Every 2–3 years, depending upon risk of exposure
Contraindications:	Severe adverse reaction to previous dose
Adverse reactions:	Minor local or systemic reactions
Before departure:	Pre-exposure prophylaxis for those planning a prolonged stay or visiting hyperendemic areas, parks and game reserves in endemic countries
Special precautions:	Avoid contact with wild and captive animals and with free-roaming animals, especially dogs and cats

TICK-BORNE ENCEPHALITIS

Disease and occurrence

See Chapter 5.

Risk for travellers

Travellers who walk and camp in infested areas during the tick season (usually spring to early autumn) are at risk and should be vaccinated. Some degree of protection is afforded by clothing that covers as much skin as possible and by applying insect repellent.

Vaccine

The vaccine should be offered only to high-risk travellers. It is an inactivated whole-cell virus vaccine containing a suspension of purified TBE virus grown on chick embryo cells and inactivated with formaldehyde. Two doses of 0.5 ml should be given i.m. 4–12 weeks apart. A third dose is given 9–12 months after the second dose, and confers immunity for 3 years. Booster doses are required to maintain immunity and should be given every 3 years if the risk continues. Outside endemic countries, the vaccine may be unlicensed and will have to be obtained by special request.

Precautions and contraindications

Occasional local reactions may occur, such as reddening and swelling around the injection site, swelling of the regional lymph nodes or general reactions (e.g. fatigue, pain in the limb, nausea and headache). Rarely, there may be fever above

38 °C for a short time, vomiting or transient rash. In very rare cases, neuritis of varying severity may be seen, although the etiological relationship to vaccination is uncertain. The vaccination has been suspected of aggravating autoimmune diseases such as multiple sclerosis and iridocyclitis, but this remains unproven. Sensitivity to thiomersal (a vaccine preservative) is a contraindication.

Type of vaccine:	Killed
Number of doses:	Two, given i.m. 4–12 weeks apart, plus booster
Booster:	9–12 months after second dose
Contraindications:	Sensitivity to the vaccine preservative thiomersal; adverse reaction to previous dose
Adverse reactions:	Local reactions occasionally; rarely fever
Before departure:	Second dose 2 weeks before departure
Recommended for:	High-risk individuals only
Special precautions:	Avoid ticks; remove immediately if bitten

TUBERCULOSIS

Disease and occurrence

See Chapter 5.

Risk for travellers

Most travellers are at low risk for tuberculosis (TB). The risk for long-term travellers (>3 months) in a country with a higher incidence of tuberculosis than their own may be comparable to the risk for local residents. Living conditions, as well as duration of travel, are important in determining the risk of infection: high-risk settings include health facilities, prisons and shelters for the homeless.

Vaccine

BCG vaccine is of very limited use for travellers. In the first year of life it provides good protection against complications of TB. In countries with high TB prevalence, infants are generally immunized as soon after birth as possible with a single dose of BCG, which protects against severe forms of TB in infancy and early childhood. Other protective benefits of the vaccine are uncertain. BCG should be considered for infants travelling from an area of low incidence to one of high incidence.

For health workers BCG provides some level of protection and one dose should be offered.

Many industrialized countries with a low incidence of TB have ceased giving BCG routinely to neonates; instead, a dose is given in adolescence. Other countries do not use BCG at all but rely on early detection and treatment to control the disease.

Booster doses of BCG are not recommended by WHO.

Precautions and contraindications

BCG is one of the more difficult vaccines to administer and the reconstituted vaccine must be given intradermally. Symptomatic HIV-infected individuals should not be vaccinated.

Type of vaccine:	Live bacterial (BCG)
Number of doses:	One
Contraindications:	Symptomatic HIV infection
Adverse reactions:	Local: abscess, regional lymphadenitis. Distant (rare): osteitis, disseminated disease
Before departure:	4 weeks
Consider for:	Infants under 6 months of age travelling to high-risk countries and health workers
Special precautions:	Skin test adults before administration; do not vaccinate if reaction is greater than 5 mm

TYPHOID FEVER

Disease and occurrence

See Chapter 5.

Risk for travellers

All travellers to endemic areas are at potential risk of typhoid fever, although the risk is generally low in tourist and business centres where standards of accommodation, sanitation and food hygiene are high. The risk is particularly high in the Indian subcontinent. Even vaccinated individuals should take care to avoid consumption of potentially contaminated food and water.

Vaccine

Travellers to countries where the risk of typhoid fever is high, especially those staying for longer than a month, those exposed to conditions of poor hygiene, and those visiting the Indian subcontinent and destinations where there is the possibility of antibiotic-resistant organisms, may be offered one of the following vaccines.

- Oral Ty21a. This live attenuated mutant strain of *Salmonella typhi* Ty21a, supplied as liquid or enteric coated capsules, is given orally in three doses (four in USA) 2 days apart, and produces protection 7 days after the final dose. Seven years after the final dose the protective efficacy is still 67% in residents of endemic areas but may be less for travellers.

- Injectable Vi CPS. Capsular Vi polysaccharide vaccine (Vi CPS), containing 25 µg of polysaccharide per dose, is given i.m. in a single dose and produces protection 7 days after injection. In endemic areas, the protective efficacy is 72% after 1.5 years and 50% 3 years after vaccination.

Both vaccines are safe and effective, currently licensed and available. They offer alternatives to the previous, poorly tolerated, whole-cell typhoid vaccine. However, their efficacy in children under 2 years of age has not been demonstrated.

A combined typhoid/hepatitis A vaccine is also available.

Precautions and contraindications

Proguanil, mefloquine and antibiotics should be stopped from 1 week (12 hours in the USA) before starting Ty21a until 1 week after.

Comparison of the adverse effects of typhoid vaccines show that more systemic reactions (e.g. fever) occur after i.m. administration of inactivated vaccine than after either Ty21a or Vi CPS. No serious adverse effects have been reported following administration of Ty 21A or Vi polysaccharide.

These vaccines are not recommended for use in infant immunization programmes: there is insufficient information on their efficacy in children under 2 years of age.

Type of vaccine:	Oral Ty21a and injectable Vi CPS
Number of doses:	One of Vi CPS, i.m. Three or four of live Ty21a, given orally at 2-day intervals as liquid or enteric coated capsule
Booster:	Every 3 years for Vi CPS, every 6 years for Ty21a
Contraindications:	Stop proguanil, mefloquine and antibiotics 1 week (12 hours in the USA) before starting Ty21a until 1 week after
Adverse reactions:	None significant
Before departure:	1 week
Recommended for:	Travellers to high-risk areas and travellers staying longer than 1 month or likely to consume food or beverages away from the usual tourist routes in developing countries
Special precautions:	Vi CPS – not under 2 years of age; avoid proguanil, mefloquine and antibiotics with Ty21a

YELLOW FEVER

Disease and occurrence

See Chapter 5.

Risk for travellers

The normally low risk to travellers increases with travel to jungle areas in endemic countries and in or near cities during urban outbreaks. Areas where yellow fever virus is present far exceed those officially reported. The risk of exposure to infection can be reduced by taking measures to prevent mosquito bites (see Chapter 3). It should be noted that the mosquito vectors of yellow fever bite mostly during daylight hours.

Vaccine

Yellow fever vaccine is highly effective (approaching 100%), while the disease may be fatal in adults who are not immune. Vaccination is recommended for all travellers (with few exceptions, see below) who visit countries or areas where there is a risk of yellow fever transmission. For domestic travel, vaccination is recommended for travel outside the urban areas of countries in the yellow fever endemic zone (Africa and south America), even if these countries have not officially reported the disease.

Note. Vaccination for personal protection of travellers is not a mandatory requirement.

Precautions and contraindications

Tolerance of the vaccine is generally excellent—only 2–5% of vaccine recipients have mild reactions, including myalgia and headache. Contraindications include true allergy to egg protein, cellular immunodeficiency (congenital or acquired, the latter sometimes being only temporary) and symptomatic HIV infection. Many industrialized countries administer yellow fever vaccine to persons with symptomatic HIV infection provided that the CD4 count is at least 400 cells/mm^3. Asymptomatic HIV-positive individuals may have a reduced response to the vaccine. There is a theoretical risk of harm to the fetus if the vaccine is given during pregnancy, but this must be weighed against the risk to the mother of remaining unvaccinated and travelling to a high-risk zone. (However, pregnant women should be advised **not** to travel to areas where exposure to yellow fever may occur.) Encephalitis has been reported as a rare event following vaccination of infants under 9 months of age; as a result, administration of the vaccine is not recommended before 9 months of age.

There have been recent reports of a small number of serious adverse reactions, including deaths, following yellow fever vaccination; most of these reactions occurred in elderly persons. However, the risk to unvaccinated individuals who visit endemic countries is far greater than the risk of a vaccine-related adverse event. It remains important for all travellers at risk to be vaccinated; nonetheless, yellow fever vaccination should not be prescribed for individuals who are not at risk of exposure to infection.

Type of vaccine:	Live viral
Number of doses:	One priming dose of 0.5 ml
Booster:	10-yearly
Contraindications:	Egg allergy; immunodeficiency from medication, disease or symptomatic HIV infection; hypersensitivity to a previous dose; pregnancy (see text above)
Adverse reactions:	Rarely, encephalitis or hepatic failure
Before departure:	International certificate of vaccination becomes valid 10 days after vaccination
Recommended for:	All travellers to endemic zones
Special precautions:	Not for infants under 9 months of age; restrictions in pregnancy

Mandatory vaccination

Yellow fever

Mandatory vaccination against yellow fever is carried out to prevent the importation of yellow fever virus into vulnerable countries. These are countries where yellow fever does not occur but where the mosquito vector and non-human primate hosts are present. Importation of the virus by an infected traveller could potentially lead to the establishment of infection in mosquitoes and primates, with a consequent risk of infection for the local population. In such cases, vaccination is an entry requirement for all travellers arriving from countries, including airport transit, where there is a risk of yellow fever transmission.

If yellow fever vaccination is contraindicated for medical reasons, a medical certificate is required for exemption.

The international yellow fever vaccination certificate becomes valid 10 days after vaccination and remains valid for a period of 10 years.

For information on countries that require proof of yellow fever vaccination as a condition of entry, see country list.

Travellers should be aware that the absence of a requirement for vaccination does *not* imply that there is no risk of exposure to yellow fever in the country.

The international certificate of vaccination is reproduced with explanatory notes on page 129.

Meningococcal meningitis

Vaccination against meningococcal meningitis is required by Saudi Arabia for all pilgrims who visit Mecca for the Umrah and Hajj. A number of countries require vaccination of travellers returning from the Umrah and Hajj.

Following the occurrence of cases of meningitis due to *N. meningitidis* W-135 among pilgrims in 2000, the current requirement is for vaccination with quadrivalent vaccine (A, C, Y and W-135). Vaccine requirements for Hajj pilgrims are issued each year and published in the *Weekly epidemiological record*.

Special groups

Infants and young children

Because not all vaccines can be administered to the very young, it is especially important to ensure protection against health hazards such as foodborne illnesses and mosquito bites by means other than vaccination. Some vaccines can be administered in the first few days of life (BCG, oral poliomyelitis vaccine, hepatitis A and B). Others (diphtheria/tetanus/pertussis, diphtheria/tetanus, inactivated poliomyelitis vaccine) should not be given before 6 weeks of age, and yellow fever vaccine not before 9 months of age. Because it may be difficult to reduce children's exposure to environmental dangers such as placing contaminated objects in the mouth or mosquito bites, it is particularly important to ensure that their routine vaccinations are fully up to date. A child who travels abroad before completing the full schedule of routine vaccines is at risk from vaccine-preventable diseases.

Adolescents and young adults

Adolescents and young adults make up the largest group of travellers and the group most likely to acquire sexually transmitted diseases. They are particularly at risk when travelling on a limited budget and using accommodation of poor standard (e.g. when backpacking), as well as from a lifestyle that may include risky sexual behaviour and other risks taken under the influence of alcohol or drugs. Because risk reduction through behaviour modification may not be reliable, this age group should be strongly encouraged to accept all appropriate vaccines before travel and to adhere to other precautions for avoiding infectious diseases.

Frequent travellers

Individuals who travel widely, usually by air, often become lax about taking precautions regarding their health. Having travelled numerous times without major health upsets, they may neglect to check that they are up to date with vaccination. Such travellers pose a special problem for health advisers who should, nonetheless, encourage compliance.

Last-minute travellers

Certain individuals, including emergency aid and health care workers, may need to travel at very short notice to dangerous, often war-torn countries. It may be difficult to give them multiple vaccines in a short space of time. If some vaccines have not been administered by the time of departure, it may be possible for the traveller to carry the doses safely in a vacuum flask (with or without ice, depending on the required temperature for the vaccine), together with the appropriate injection devices. Vaccines should travel well like this until they can be stored at the appropriate temperature at the destination, awaiting timely use. If there is any doubt about being able to keep vaccines cold in transit, the traveller should be encouraged to obtain the remaining doses in the country of destination after the appropriate interval.

Those in occupations that make the need for emergency travel likely to arise should be strongly encouraged to keep their routine and other recommended vaccinations fully up to date.

Pregnancy

Pregnancy should not deter a woman from receiving vaccines that are safe and will protect both her health and that of her child. However, care must be taken to avoid the inappropriate administration of certain vaccines that could harm

Table 6.2 **Vaccination in pregnancy**

Vaccine		Use in pregnancy	Comments
BCG[a]		No	
Cholera			Safety not determined
Hepatitis A		Yes, administer if indicated	Safety not determined
Hepatitis B		Yes, administer if indicated	
Influenza		Yes, administer if indicated	In some circumstances—consult a physician
Japanese encephalitis			Safety not determined
Measles[a]		No	
Meningococcal disease		Yes, administer if indicated	
Mumps[a]		No	
Poliomyelitis	OPV	Yes, administer if indicated	
	IPV	Yes, administer if indicated	Normally avoided
Rubella[a]		No	
Tetanus/diphtheria		Yes, administer if indicated	
Rabies		Yes, administer if indicated	
Typhoid Ty21a			Safety not determined
Varicella[a]		No	
Yellow fever[a]		Yes, administer if indicated	Avoided unless at high risk

[a] Live vaccine—to be avoided during pregnancy.

the unborn baby. Killed or inactivated vaccines, toxoids and polysaccharides can generally be given during pregnancy, as can oral polio vaccine. Live vaccines are generally contraindicated because of largely theoretical risks to the baby. Measles, mumps, rubella, BCG and yellow fever vaccines should be avoided in pregnancy. The risks and benefits should nevertheless be examined in each individual case. Vaccination against yellow fever may be considered after the sixth month of pregnancy when the risk from exposure is deemed greater than the risk to the fetus (see Table 6.2). However, pregnant women should be advised *not* to travel to areas where there is a risk of exposure to yellow fever.

Elderly travellers

Vaccination of healthy elderly travellers does not differ in principle from vaccination of younger adults. However, special considerations arise if the elderly traveller has not been fully immunized in the past and/or has existing medical problems.

Many elderly people may have never been vaccinated with the vaccines used in routine childhood immunization programmes, or may have neglected to keep up the recommended schedule of booster doses. As a consequence, they may be susceptible to diseases such as diphtheria, tetanus and poliomyelitis as well as to other infections present at the travel destination.

Elderly travellers who have never been vaccinated should be offered a full primary course of vaccination against diphtheria, tetanus, poliomyelitis and hepatitis B. In addition, those who are not immune to hepatitis A should be vaccinated against this disease before travelling to a developing country.

Since the elderly are at risk for severe and complicated influenza, regular annual vaccination is recommended. For travellers from one hemisphere to the other, vaccine against the currently circulating strains of influenza is unlikely to be obtainable before arrival at the travel destination. Those arriving shortly before, or early during, the influenza season, and planning to stay for more than 2–3 weeks, should arrange vaccination as soon as possible after arrival. Pneumococcal vaccine should also be considered for elderly travellers in view of the risk of pneumococcal pneumonia following influenza infection.

Special considerations arise in the case of elderly travellers with pre-existing chronic health problems (see below).

Travellers with chronic medical problems

Travellers with chronic medical conditions involving impaired immunity, including cancer, diabetes mellitus, HIV infection and treatment with immunosuppressive drugs, may be at risk of severe complications following administration of vaccines that contain live organisms. Consequently, it may be advisable to avoid measles, oral polio, yellow fever and BCG vaccines for these travellers. For travel to a country where yellow fever vaccination is mandatory, a medical certificate will be required to obtain exemption.

Travellers with chronic cardiovascular and/or respiratory conditions or diabetes mellitus are at high risk for severe influenza and its complications. Regular annual vaccination against influenza is recommended. For travel from one hemisphere to the other shortly before, or early, during the influenza season, vaccination should be sought as soon as possible after arrival at the travel destination (see also pages 102–103).

For those who lack a functional spleen, additional vaccines are advised: Hib, meningococcal vaccine (conjugate C as well as A+C or quadrivalent vaccine) and pneumococcal vaccination should be considered, in addition to regular vaccination against influenza.

HIV-positive and immunocompromised travellers

The likelihood of successful immunization is reduced in some HIV-infected children and adults, but the risk of serious adverse effects remains low. Asymptomatic HIV-infected children should be immunized according to standard schedules. With certain exceptions, symptomatic HIV-positive individuals should also be immunized as usual. Both measles and oral poliomyelitis vaccines may be given to persons with symptomatic HIV infection. The following are contraindicated for this group:

- *Measles vaccine* has generally been recommended for individuals with moderate immunodeficiency if there is even a low risk of contracting wild measles from the community. A low level of risk is associated with use of measles vaccine in individuals who are HIV-infected and whose immune system is impaired. Where the risk of contracting wild measles infection is negligible, it may be preferable to avoid use of the vaccine.

- *Yellow fever vaccine* is not recommended for symptomatic HIV-positive adults and children. It is not certain whether yellow fever vaccine poses a risk for asymptomatic HIV-infected persons. Any adverse reactions to the vaccine occurring in HIV-positive individuals should be reported to WHO. In many industrialized countries, yellow fever vaccine is administered to people with symptomatic HIV infection or suffering from other immunodeficiency diseases, provided that their CD4 count is at least 400 cells/mm^3 and if they plan to visit areas where epidemic or endemic yellow fever actually occurs.

- *BCG vaccine* should not be given to individuals with symptomatic HIV/AIDS.

Adverse reactions and contraindications

Reactions to vaccines

While vaccines are generally both effective and safe, no vaccine is totally safe for all recipients. Vaccination may sometimes cause certain mild side-effects: local reaction, slight fever and other systemic symptoms may develop as part of the normal immune response. In addition, certain components of the vaccine (e.g. aluminium adjuvant, antibiotics or preservatives) occasionally cause reactions. A successful vaccine reduces these reactions to a minimum while inducing maximum immunity. Serious reactions are rare. Health workers who administer vaccines have an obligation to inform recipients of known adverse reactions and the likelihood of their occurrence.

A known contraindication should be clearly marked on a traveller's vaccination card, so that the vaccine may be avoided in future. In exceptional circumstances, the medical adviser may consider the risk of a particular disease to be greater than the theoretical risk of administering the vaccine and will advise vaccination.

Common mild vaccine reactions

Most vaccines produce some mild local and/or systemic reactions (summarized in Table 6.3) relatively frequently. These reactions generally occur within a day or two of immunization. However, the systemic symptoms that may arise with measles or MMR vaccine occur 5–12 days after vaccination. Fever and/or rash occur in 5–15% of measles/MMR vaccine recipients during this time, but only 3% are attributable to the vaccine; the rest may be classed as background events, i.e. normal events of childhood.

Uncommon, severe adverse reactions

Most of the rare vaccine reactions (detailed in Table 6.4) are self-limiting and do not lead to long-term problems. Anaphylaxis, for example, although potentially fatal, can be treated and has no long-term effects.

Encephalopathy is included as a rare reaction to measles or DTP vaccine, but there is no certainty that there is a causal relationship.

Although extremely rare, a reaction to yellow fever vaccine can be life-threatening and unpredictable. Ideally, anyone who receives the vaccine should be asked to stay in the clinic for 15–30 minutes; if a reaction occurs, it can be treated and potentially serious consequences avoided.

All serious reactions should be reported immediately to the relevant national health authority and marked on the vaccination card. In addition, the patient and relatives should be instructed to avoid the vaccination in the future.

Table 6.3 **Summary of common minor vaccine reactions**

Vaccine	Possible minor adverse reaction	Expected frequency
BCG	Local reaction (pain, swelling, redness)	Common
Cholera	Oral presentation—none	
DTP	Local reaction (pain, swelling, redness)	Up to 50%[a]
	Fever	Up to 50%
Hepatitis A	Local reaction (pain, swelling, redness)	Up to 50%
Hepatitis B	Local reaction (pain, swelling, redness)	Adults up to 30%, Children up to 5%
	Fever	1–6%
Hib	Local reaction (pain, swelling, redness)	5–15%
	Fever	2–10%
Japanese encephalitis	Local reaction, low-grade fever, myalgia, gastrointestinal upset	Up to 20%
Lyme disease	Local reaction, myalgia, influenza-like illness	Up to 20%
Measles/MMR	Local reaction (pain, swelling, redness) Irritability, malaise and non-specific symptoms, fever	Up to 10% Up to 5%
Pneumococcal	Local reaction (pain, swelling, redness)	30–50%
Poliomyelitis (OPV)	None	Less than 1%
Poliomyelitis (IPV)	None	
Rabies	Local and/or general reaction depending on type of vaccine (see product information)	15–25%

Vaccine	Possible minor adverse reaction	Expected frequency
Meningococcal	Mild local reactions	Up to 71%
Tetanus/Td	Local reaction (pain, swelling, redness)[b]	Up to 10%
	Malaise and non-specific symptoms	Up to 25%
Tick-borne encephalitis	Local reaction (pain, swelling, redness)	Up to 10%
Typhoid fever	Depends on type of vaccine use (see product information)	—
Yellow fever	Headache	10%
	Influenza-like symptoms	22%
	Local reaction (pain, swelling, redness)	5%

[a] With whole-cell pertussis vaccine. Rates for acellular pertussis vaccine are lower.
[b] Rate of local reactions likely to increase with booster doses, up to 50–85%.

Table 6.4 **Uncommon severe adverse reactions**

Vaccine	Possible adverse reaction[a]	Expected rate per million doses[b]
BCG	Suppurative lymphadenitis	100–1000
	BCG-osteitis	1–700
	Disseminated BCG-itis	2
Cholera	NR	—
DTP	Persistent crying	1000–60 000
	Seizures	570
	Hypotonic–hyporesponsive episode	570
	Anaphylaxis	20
Hepatitis A	NR	—
Hepatitis B[c]	Anaphylaxis	1–2
	Guillain–Barré syndrome (plasma-derived)	5
Hib	NR	—
Japanese encephalitis	Mouse-brain only—neurological event	Rare
	Hypersensitivity	100–6400
Lyme disease	NR	—

Vaccine	Possible adverse reaction[a]	Expected rate per million doses[b]
Measles/MMR	Febrile seizure	333
	Thrombocytopenic purpura	33–45
	Anaphylaxis	1–50
	Encephalitis	1
Meningococcal	Anaphylaxis	1
Mumps	Depends on strain—aseptic meningitis	0–500
Pneumococcal	Anaphylaxis	Very rare
Poliomyelitis (OPV)	Vaccine-associated paralytic poliomyelitis	1.4–3.4
Poliomyelitis (IPV)	NR	—
Rabies	Animal brain tissue only—neuroparalysis	17–44
Rubella	Arthralgia/arthritis/arthropathy	None or very rare
Tetanus	Brachial neuritis	5–10
	Anaphylaxis	1–6
Tick-borne encephalitis	NR	—
Typhoid fever	Parenteral vaccine—various	Very rare
	Oral vaccine—NR	—
Yellow fever	Encephalitis	500–4000 (<6 months)
	Allergy/anaphylaxis	5–20
	Hepatic failure	Rare

[a] NR = none reported.
[b] Precise rate may vary with survey method.
[c] Although there have been anecdotal reports of demyelinating disease following hepatitis B vaccine, there is no scientific evidence for a causal relationship.

Contraindications

The main contraindications to the administration of vaccines are summarized in Table 6.5.

Table 6.5 **Contraindications to vaccines**

Vaccine	Contraindications
All	A severe adverse event following a dose of vaccine (e.g. anaphylaxis,[a] encephalitis/encephalopathy, or non-febrile convulsions) is a true contraindication to further immunization with the antigen concerned and a subsequent dose should not be given. Current serious illness.
Live vaccines (MMR, BCG, yellow fever)	Pregnancy. Radiation therapy (i.e. total-body radiation).
Yellow fever	Egg allergy. Immunodeficiency (from medication, disease or symptomatic HIV infection[b]).
BCG	Symptomatic HIV infection.
Influenza, yellow fever	History of anaphylactic reactions[a] following egg ingestion. No vaccines prepared in hen's egg tissues (i.e. yellow fever and influenza vaccines) should be given. (Vaccine viruses propagated in chicken fibroblast cells, e.g. measles or MMR vaccines, can usually be given however.)
Pertussis-containing vaccines	A serious reaction to a dose of DTP. The pertussis component should be omitted for subsequent doses and diphtheria and tetanus immunization completed with DT vaccine. Evolving neurological disease (e.g. uncontrolled epilepsy or progressive encephalopathy). Vaccines containing the whole-cell pertussis component should not be given to children with this problem. Acellular vaccine is less reactogenic and is used in many industrialized countries instead of whole-cell pertussis vaccine.

[a] Generalized urticaria, difficulty in breathing, swelling of the mouth and throat, hypotension or shock.

[b] In many industrialized countries yellow fever vaccine is administered to individuals with symptomatic HIV infection or who are suffering from other immunodeficiency diseases, provided that their CD4 count is at least 400 cells/mm^3 and if they plan to visit areas where epidemic or endemic yellow fever actually occurs.

Further reading

WHO information on vaccine preventable diseases: http://www.who.int/vaccines/

Global Influenza Surveillance Network (FluNet): http://oms2.b3e.jussieu.fr/flunet/

International certificate of vaccination

The certificate must be *printed* in English and French; an additional language may be added. It must be *completed* in English or French; an additional language may be used.

The international certificate of vaccination is an *individual* certificate. It should not be used collectively. Separate certificates should be issued for children; the information should not be incorporated in the mother's certificate.

An international certificate is valid only if the yellow fever vaccine used has been approved by WHO and if the vaccinating centre has been designated by the national health administration for the area in which the centre is situated. The date should be recorded in the following sequence: day, month, year, with the month written in letters, e.g. 8 January 2001.

A certificate issued to a child who is unable to write should be signed by a parent or guardian. For illiterates, the signature should be indicated by their mark certified by another person.

Although a nurse may carry out the vaccination under the direct supervision of a qualified medical practitioner, the certificate must be signed by the person authorized by the national health administration. The official stamp of the centre is not an accepted substitute for a personal signature.

> *Signature of person vaccinated*
> *Signature de la personne vaccinée*

> *e.g.: 8 January 2001*
> *ex.: 8 janvier 2001*

> *Signature required*
> *(rubber stamp not accepted)*
> *Signature exigée (le cachet*
> *n'est pas suffisant)*

> *Official stamp*
> *Cachet officiel*

WHO 881091

International certificate of vaccination or revaccination against yellow fever
Certificat international de vaccination ou de revaccination contre la fièvre jaune

| is to certify that
ussigné(e) certifie que | Ole OLSEN | | date of birth
né(e) le | 8 Nov.
1945 | sex
sexe | M |

e signature follows ___C. Olsen___
la signature suit

n the date indicated been vaccinated or revaccinated against yellow fever.
vacciné(e) ou revacciné(e) contre la fièvre jaune à la date indiquée.

Date	Signature and professional status of vaccinator Signature et titre du vaccinateur	Manufacturer and batch no. of vaccine Fabricant du vaccin et numéro du lot	Official stamp of vaccinating centre Cachet officiel du centre de vaccination
8 January 2001	Dr John Doe M.D.	R.I.V. 63007	

This certificate is valid only if the vaccine used has been approved by the World Health Organization and if the vaccinating centre has been designated by the health administration for the territory in which that centre is situated.

The validity of this certificate shall extend for a period of 10 years, beginning 10 days after the date of vaccination or, in the event of a revaccination within such period of 10 years, from the date of that revaccination.

This certificate must be signed in his own hand by a medical practitioner or other person authorized by the national health administration; an official stamp is not an accepted substitute for a signature.

Any amendment of this certificate, or erasure, or failure to complete any part of it, may render it invalid.

Ce certificat n'est valable que si le vaccin employé a été approuvé par l'Organisation mondiale de la Santé et si le centre de vaccination a été habilité par l'administration sanitaire du territoire dans lequel ce centre est situé.

La validité de ce certificat couvre une période de 10 ans commençant 10 jours après la date de la vaccination ou, dans le cas d'une revaccination au cours de cette période de 10 ans, le jour de cette revaccination.

Ce certificat doit être signé de sa propre main par un médecin ou une autre personne habilitée par l'administration sanitaire nationale, un cachet officiel ne pouvant être considéré comme tenant lieu de signature.

Toute correction ou rature sur le certificat ou l'omission d'une quelconque des mentions qu'il comporte peut affecter sa validité.

CHAPTER 7

Malaria

General considerations

Malaria is a common and life-threatening disease in many tropical and subtropical areas. It is currently endemic in over 100 countries, which are visited by more than 125 million international travellers every year.

Each year many international travellers fall ill with malaria while visiting countries where the disease is endemic, and well over 10 000 fall ill after returning home. Fever occurring in a traveller within two to three months of leaving a malaria-endemic area is a medical emergency and should be investigated urgently.

Cause

Human malaria is caused by four different species of the protozoan parasite *Plasmodium*: *Plasmodium falciparum*, *P. vivax*, *P. ovale* and *P. malariae*.

Transmission

The malaria parasite is transmitted by various species of *Anopheles* mosquitoes, which bite mainly between sunset and sunrise.

Nature of the disease

Malaria is an acute febrile illness with an incubation period of 7 days or longer. Thus, a febrile illness developing less than one week after the first possible exposure is not malaria.

The most severe form is caused by *P. falciparum*, in which variable clinical features include fever, chills, headache, muscular aching and weakness, vomiting, cough, diarrhoea and abdominal pain; other symptoms related to organ failure may supervene, followed by coma and death. The initial symptoms, which may be mild, may not be easy to recognize as being due to malaria. It is important that the possibility of falciparum malaria is considered in all cases of unexplained fever starting at any time between the seventh day of first possible exposure to malaria and two months (or, rarely, later) after the last possible exposure, and any individual who experiences a fever in this interval should immediately seek diagnosis and effective treatment.

Early diagnosis and appropriate treatment can be life-saving. Falciparum malaria may be fatal if treatment is delayed beyond 24 hours. A blood sample should be examined for malaria parasites. If no parasites are found in the first blood film but symptoms persist, a series of blood samples should be taken and examined at 6–12-hour intervals. Other early symptoms of infection may include headache, muscular aching and weakness, vomiting, diarrhoea and cough.

Pregnant women and young children are particularly susceptible to severe and complicated falciparum malaria. Malaria in pregnant travellers increases the risk of maternal death, miscarriage, stillbirth and neonatal death.

The forms of malaria caused by other *Plasmodium* species are less severe and rarely life-threatening.

The malaria situation is becoming worse in many areas. Prevention and treatment of falciparum malaria is becoming more difficult because *P. falciparum* is increasingly resistant to various antimalarial drugs. Of the other malaria species, drug resistance has to date only been reported for *P. vivax*, mainly from Indonesia (Irian Jaya) and Papua New Guinea, with more sporadic cases reported from Brazil, Guatemala, Guyana, India and Myanmar.

Geographical distribution

The current distribution of malaria in the world is shown in the map on page 80. Affected countries and territories are listed on page 148.

In many endemic countries of central and south America, Asia and the Mediterranean region, the main urban areas—but not necessarily the outskirts of towns—are free of malaria transmission. However, malaria can occur in main urban areas in Africa and India. There is usually less risk of the disease at altitudes above 1500 metres, but in favourable climatic conditions it can occur at altitudes up to almost 3000 metres. The risk of infection may also vary according to the season, being highest at the end of the rainy season.

There may be no risk of malaria in many tourist destinations in south-east Asia and Latin America.

Risk for travellers

During the transmission season in malaria-endemic areas, all non-immune travellers exposed to mosquito bites, especially between dusk and dawn, are at risk of clinical malaria. Most cases of malaria in travellers occur because of poor compliance with prophylactic drug regimens or use of inappropriate prophylaxis.

Falciparum malaria can be fatal, and it is estimated that about 1% of patients with *P. falciparum* infection die of the disease. Young children, pregnant women and elderly travellers are at increased risk. The most important factors that determine the survival of patients with *P. falciparum* infection are early diagnosis and appropriate treatment.

Travellers to countries where the degree of malaria transmission varies in different areas should be advised of the risk of malaria in the specific zones that they will be visiting. If specific information is not available before travelling, it is recommended to assume that there is a uniformly high malaria risk throughout the country. This applies particularly to individuals backpacking to remote places and visiting areas where diagnostic facilities and medical care are not readily available. Travellers staying overnight in rural areas may be at highest risk.

Precautions

Travellers and their advisers should note the four principles of malaria protection:

— Be aware of the risk, the incubation period, and the main symptoms.

— Avoid being bitten by mosquitoes, especially between dusk and dawn.

— Take antimalarial drugs (chemoprophylaxis) to suppress infection where appropriate.

— Immediately seek diagnosis and treatment if a fever develops one week or more after entering an area where there is a malaria risk.

Personal protection against mosquito bites is the first line of defence against malaria; protective measures are described in Chapter 3. In addition, travellers should take chemoprophylaxis where appropriate.

Chemoprophylaxis

The correct dosage of the most appropriate antimalarial drug(s) (if any) for the destination(s) should be prescribed (see country list and Table 7.1). The following should also be taken into account:

- Dosing schedules for children should be based on body weight.
- Antimalarials that have to be taken daily should be started the day before arrival in the risk area.
- Weekly chloroquine should be started 1 week before arrival.
- Weekly mefloquine should be started at least 1 week, but preferably 2–3 weeks before departure, to provide optimal protective blood levels and to allow any side-effects to be detected before travel so that possible alternatives can be considered.
- Antimalarial drugs must be taken with food and swallowed with plenty of water.
- All prophylactic drugs should be taken with unfailing regularity for the duration of the stay in the malaria risk area, and should be continued for 4 weeks after the last possible exposure to infection, since parasites may still emerge from the liver during this period. The single exception is atovaquone/proguanil, which can be stopped 1 week after return.
- No antimalarial prophylactic regimen provides complete protection.
- Precautions to avoid mosquito bites are necessary even when antimalarial drugs are taken.

Depending on the area visited (see country list) the recommended prophylaxis may be chloroquine, chloroquine plus proguanil, mefloquine or doxycycline. In areas where mefloquine is the prophylactic drug of choice, doxycycline can be used as an alternative; chloroquine plus proguanil would offer less protection. Chloroquine on its own can be recommended only for areas where malaria is due exclusively to *P. vivax* or where there is a low risk of chloroquine-sensitive *P. falciparum*.

Atovaquone/proguanil offers an alternative prophylaxis for travellers who are making short trips to areas where there is chloroquine resistance, and who cannot take mefloquine or doxycycline. It is registered in 11 European countries for chemoprophylactic use, with a restriction on body weight (> 40 kg) and duration of use (no more than 28 days). In the USA these restrictions do not apply. See Table 7.2 for details on individual drugs.

All antimalarial drugs have specific contraindications and possible side-effects. Adverse reactions attributed to malaria chemoprophylaxis are common, but most are minor and do not affect the activities of the traveller. Serious adverse events — defined as constituting an apparent threat to life, requiring or prolonging hospitalization, or resulting in severe disability—are rare. With mefloquine the incidence range of serious adverse events has been estimated at 1 per 6000 to 1 per 10 600 travellers, compared with 1 per 13 600 with chloroquine. The risk associated with the drug should be weighed against the risk of malaria, especially falciparum malaria, and local drug-resistance patterns.

Each of the antimalarial drugs is contraindicated in certain groups and individuals, and the contraindications should be carefully considered (see Table 7.2) to reduce the risk of serious adverse reactions. In case of doubt, and when only less effective alternatives are available, travellers should start prophylaxis early (2–3 weeks before departure) to check the outcome. People with chronic illnesses should seek individual medical advice. Any traveller who develops serious side-effects to an antimalarial should stop taking the drug and seek immediate medical attention. This applies particularly to neurological or psychological disturbances after mefloquine and to rashes after sulfadoxine–pyrimethamine treatment. Mild nausea, occasional vomiting or loose stools should not prompt discontinuation of prophylaxis, but medical advice should be sought if symptoms persist.

Because of the risk of adverse side-effects, chemoprophylaxis should not be prescribed in the absence of malaria risk. It is important to note that malaria is not present in all tropical countries (see page 148 and country list).

Long-term use of chemoprophylaxis

The risk of serious side-effects associated with long-term prophylactic use of chloroquine and proguanil is low. However, anyone who has taken 300 mg of chloroquine weekly for over five years and requires further prophylaxis should be screened twice-yearly for early retinal changes. If daily doses of 100 mg chloroquine have been taken, screening should start after three years. An alternative drug should be prescribed if changes are seen. Data indicate no increased risk of serious side-effects with long-term use of mefloquine. Experience with doxycycline for long-term chemoprophylaxis (i.e. more than 4–6 months) is limited, but available data are reassuring. Mefloquine and doxycycline should be reserved for those at greatest risk of chloroquine-resistant infections. Atovaquone/proguanil cannot be recommended for long-term chemo-prophylactic use because of the lack of data; European countries have restricted its use to 28 days.

Stand-by emergency treatment

An individual who experiences a fever 1 week or more after entering an area of malaria risk should consult a physician or qualified malaria laboratory immediately to obtain diagnosis and treatment. Most travellers will be able to obtain medical attention within 24 hours of the onset of fever. For a minority, however, this may be impossible, particularly if they will be staying (1 week or more after entering an endemic area) in a remote location. In such cases, travellers are advised to carry antimalarial drugs for self-administration ("stand-by emergency treatment"). The choice of drugs for stand-by emergency treatments in relation to the drugs used for prophylaxis is given in Table 7.1.

Stand-by emergency treatment may also be indicated for travellers in some occupational groups, such as aircraft crews, who make frequent short stops in endemic areas over a prolonged period of time. Such travellers may eventually choose to reserve chemoprophylaxis for high-risk areas only. However, they should continue to take rigorous measures for protection against mosquito bites and be prepared for an attack of malaria: they should always carry a course of antimalarial drugs for stand-by emergency treatment, seek immediate medical care in case of fever, and take stand-by emergency treatment if prompt medical help is not available.

Stand-by emergency treatment—combined with rigorous protection against mosquito bites—may occasionally be indicated for those who travel for 1 week or more to remote rural areas where there is a very low likelihood of multidrug-resistant malaria and the risk of side-effects of prophylaxis outweighs the risk of contracting malaria. This may be the case in certain border areas of countries in south-east Asia where the risk of side-effects may outweigh the risk of becoming infected. However, most travellers to these areas will be able to access competent medical care within 24 hours of the onset of fever.

Studies on the use of rapid diagnostic tests ("dipsticks") have shown that untrained travellers experience major problems in the performance and interpretation of these tests, with an unacceptably high number of false-negative results. Major technical modifications are required before dipsticks can be recommended for use by travellers.

Travellers provided with stand-by emergency treatment should be given clear and precise written instructions on the recognition of symptoms, when and how to take the treatment, the treatment regimen, possible side-effects, and the possibility of drug failure. They should be made aware that self-treatment is a first-aid measure, and that they should seek medical advice as soon as possible.

In general, travellers carrying stand-by emergency treatment should observe the following guidelines:

- Consult a physician immediately if fever occurs 1 week or more after entering an area with malaria risk.

- If it is impossible to consult a physician and/or establish a diagnosis within 24 hours of the onset of fever, start the stand-by emergency treatment and seek medical care as soon as possible for complete evaluation and to exclude other serious causes of fever.

- Complete the stand-by treatment course and resume antimalarial prophylaxis 1 week after the *first* treatment dose. Mefloquine prophylaxis, however, should be resumed 1 week after the *last* treatment dose of quinine.

- Vomiting of antimalarial drugs is less likely if fever is first lowered with antipyretics. A second full dose should be taken if vomiting occurs within 30 minutes of taking the drug. If vomiting occurs 30–60 minutes after a dose, an additional half-dose should be taken. Vomiting with diarrhoea may lead to treatment failure because of poor drug absorption.

Depending on the area visited and the chemoprophylaxis regimen taken, one of the following stand-by treatment regimens can be recommended.

Chloroquine

Adults: 1500 mg chloroquine base total, taken as 6 tablets of 100 mg, followed by 6 tablets 24 hours later, and 3 tablets 48 hours after the first dose.

Children: a total dose of 25 mg chloroquine base per kg body weight over 3 days, taken as 10 mg per kg on the first and second day, and 5 mg per kg on the third day.

Sulfadoxine–pyrimethamine

Adults: single dose of 3 tablets, each containing 500 mg sulfadoxine plus 25 mg pyrimethamine.

Children: single dose of 25 mg sulfadoxine plus 1.25 mg pyrimethamine per kg body weight.

Mefloquine

15 mg base/kg (single dose) or 25 mg base/kg (split dose) depending on the extent of mefloquine resistance in the area concerned.

Adults: single dose: 4 tablets of 250 mg mefloquine;

or   split dose: 4 tablets of 250 mg mefloquine followed by 2 tablets of 250 mg mefloquine 6–24 hours later.

Children: single dose: 15 mg mefloquine base per kg body weight;

or   split dose: 15 mg mefloquine base per kg body weight followed by 10 mg base per kg body weight 6–24 hours later.

Mefloquine is contraindicated during the first 3 months of pregnancy and in infants weighing less than 5 kg.

Quinine

Adults: 2 tablets of 300 mg quinine, 3 times daily, at 8-hour intervals, for 7 days.

Children: 8 mg quinine base per kg body weight, 3 times daily, for 7 days.

Quinine plus doxycycline

Adults: quinine as above, plus doxycycline for 7 days: 2 tablets of 100 mg doxycycline salt on the first day, 12 hours apart, and 1 tablet daily for the next 6 days.

Children 8 years and older: quinine as above, plus doxycycline treatment for 7 days based on body weight: 25–35 kg, $^1/_2$ adult dose; 36–50 kg, $^3/_4$ adult dose.

Doxycycline is contraindicated during pregnancy and lactation, and in children under 8 years of age.

Note. For specific drug contraindications, see Table 7.3.

Artemether/lumefantrine has been registered for stand-by emergency treatment in Switzerland only.

Halofantrine is no longer recommended for stand-by treatment following reports that it can result in ventricular dysrhythmias and prolongation of Q–T intervals in susceptible individuals. These changes may be accentuated if halofantrine is taken with other antimalarial drugs that may reduce myocardial conduction.

Treatment of *P. vivax*, *P. ovale* and *P. malariae* infections

P. vivax and *P. ovale* can remain quiescent in the liver for many months. Relapses caused by the persistent liver forms may appear months, and rarely up to 1–2 years, after exposure. They are not prevented by current chemoprophylactic regimens. Relapses can be treated with chloroquine (or mefloquine or quinine if resistance is suspected) and further relapses prevented by a course of primaquine, which eliminates any remaining parasite in the liver. In patients with known or suspected glucose-6-phosphate dehydrogenase (G6PD) deficiency, expert medical advice should be sought since primaquine may cause haemolysis in G6PD-deficient patients. Where possible, G6PD deficiency should be excluded before antirelapse therapy with primaquine is given. Blood infection with *P. malariae* may be present for many years, but it is not life-threatening and is easily cured by a standard treatment course of chloroquine.

Special groups

Some groups of travellers, especially young children and pregnant women, are at particular risk of serious consequences if they become infected with malaria.

Pregnant women

Malaria in a pregnant woman increases the risk of maternal death, miscarriage, stillbirth and low birth weight with associated risk of neonatal death.

Pregnant women should be advised to **avoid** travelling to areas where chloroquine-resistant *P. falciparum* occurs. When travel cannot be avoided, it is very important to take effective preventive measures against malaria, even when travelling to areas with transmission of vivax malaria only.

Pregnant women should be extra diligent in using measures to protect against mosquito bites, but should take care not to exceed the recommended dosage of insect repellents.

In the few areas with exclusively *P. vivax* transmission or where *P. falciparum* can be expected to be 100% sensitive to chloroquine, prophylaxis with chloroquine alone may be used. In areas with chloroquine-resistant *P. falciparum*, prophylaxis with chloroquine plus proguanil is recommended during the first three months of pregnancy. Mefloquine prophylaxis may be given during the second and the third trimesters. Other drugs are either dangerous to the fetus or have been insufficiently well investigated to be prescribed for prophylaxis in pregnancy.

Pregnant women should seek medical help immediately if malaria is suspected; if this is not possible, they should take emergency stand-by treatment with quinine. Medical help *must* be sought as soon as possible after stand-by treatment.

Pregnant women with falciparum malaria may rapidly develop any of the clinical symptoms of severe malaria. They are particularly susceptible to hypoglycaemia and pulmonary oedema. They may develop postpartum haemorrhage, and hyperpyrexia leading to fetal distress. Any pregnant woman with severe falciparum malaria should be transferred to intensive care, and managed in close collaboration between infectious disease, internal medicine and obstetric care specialists. Because of the risk of quinine-induced hyperinsulinaemia and hypoglycaemia, artesunate and artemether are the drugs of choice for treatment of severe malaria in the second and third trimester. Data on the use of artemisinin derivatives in the first trimester are still limited.

Women who may become pregnant during or after travel

Both mefloquine and doxycycline prophylaxis may be taken, but pregnancy should be avoided during the period of drug intake and for 3 months after mefloquine and 1 week after doxycycline prophylaxis is stopped.

If pregnancy occurs during antimalarial prophylaxis, the woman's doctor should give information about the possible effects of the drugs on the fetus. However, in the case of unplanned pregnancy, malaria chemoprophylaxis is not considered to be an indication for pregnancy termination.

Young children

Falciparum malaria in a young child is a medical emergency—it may be rapidly fatal. Early symptoms are atypical and difficult to recognize, but life-threatening complications can occur within hours of the initial symptoms.

Parents should be advised **not** to take babies or young children to areas with transmission of chloroquine-resistant *P. falciparum*. If travel cannot be avoided, children must be very carefully protected against mosquito bites and be given appropriate chemoprophylactic drugs. Babies should be kept under insecticide-treated mosquito nets as much as possible between dusk and dawn. The manufacturer's instructions on the use of insect repellents should be followed diligently, and the recommended dosage must not be exceeded.

Breastfed, as well as bottle-fed, babies, should be given chemoprophylaxis since they are not protected by the mother's prophylaxis. Dosage schedules for children should be based on body weight. Chloroquine and proguanil are safe for babies and young children, and mefloquine may be given to infants of more than 5 kg body weight. Doxycycline, however, is contraindicated in children below 8 years of age and atovaquone/proguanil cannot be recommended for prophylaxis in children weighing less than 11 kg because of the lack of data.

All antimalarial drugs should be kept out of the reach of children and stored in childproof containers. Chloroquine is particularly toxic to children in case of overdose.

Medical help should be sought immediately if a child develops a febrile illness. Malaria should always be suspected and laboratory diagnosis is essential. In infants, malaria should be suspected even in non-febrile illness.

The possibility of malaria should be considered whenever a child develops a fever within a year of travelling to or immigrating from an endemic area. Laboratory diagnosis should be requested immediately if malaria is suspected, and treatment with an effective antimalarial drug initiated as soon as possible.

Special situations—multidrug-resistant malaria

In border areas between Cambodia, Myanmar and Thailand, *P. falciparum* infections do not respond to treatment with chloroquine or sulfadoxine–pyrimethamine, and sensitivity to quinine is reduced. Treatment failures in excess of 50% with mefloquine are also being reported. In these situations, doxycycline can be used for chemoprophylaxis together with rigorous personal protection measures. However, the drug is contraindicated in pregnant women and children under the age of 8 years. Since there is no prophylactic regimen that is both effective and safe for these groups in areas of multidrug-resistant malaria, pregnant women and young children should avoid travelling to these malarious areas.

The national authorities in Thailand recommend a combination of mefloquine plus artesunate or artemether as the first-line treatment in areas of highly mefloquine-resistant malaria. When these drugs are not available, infections with *P. falciparum* acquired on the Thailand/Cambodia and Thailand/Myanmar borders may be treated with a total dose of 25 mg/kg mefloquine, given as 15 mg/kg initially followed by 10 mg/kg 6–8 hours later, or with oral quinine, 10 mg/kg of body weight every 8 hours for 7 days, in combination with either tetracycline or doxycycline. In the Amazon basin of south America, mefloquine resistance has been reported only from Brazil, where clinical failure rates remain below 5%.

Table 7.1 **Choice of stand-by treatment according to recommended chemoprophylactic regimen**

Note 1. The choice of drug to be used for stand-by treatment depends on the prophylaxis taken and on the presence of drug-resistant malaria in the countries to be visited (see country list). The drug selected for stand-by treatment should be one to which no resistance has been reported in the countries concerned.

Note 2. No stand-by treatment can be recommended for travellers taking atovaquone/proguanil prophylaxis because of the lack of data and the possibility of drug interactions.

Prophylactic regimen	Stand-by treatment
None	Chloroquine, for *P. vivax* areas only
	Sulfadoxine–pyrimethamine combination
	Mefloquine, 15 mg/kg
	Quinine
Chloroquine alone or with proguanil	Sulfadoxine–pyrimethamine combination
	Mefloquine, 15 mg/kg
	Quinine
Mefloquine	Sulfadoxine–pyrimethamine combination
	Quinine[a]
	Quinine + doxycycline/tetracycline for 7 days[a]
Doxycycline	Mefloquine, 25 mg/kg
	Quinine + tetracycline for 7 days

[a] In these situations, mefloquine prophylaxis should only be resumed 7 days after the last self-treatment dose of quinine.

Further reading

Management of severe malaria: a practical handbook, 2nd ed. Geneva, WHO, 2000.

WHO Expert Committee on Malaria. Twentieth report. WHO, Geneva, 2000 (WHO Technical Report Series, No. 892).

The use of antimalarial drugs (2001): http://whqlibdoc.who.int/hq/2001/WHO_CDS_RBM_2001.33.pdf

Table 7.2 **Use of antimalarial drugs for prophylaxis in travellers**

Generic name	Dosage regimen	Duration of prophylaxis	Use in special groups			Contraindications	Comments
			Pregnancy	Breast-feeding	Children		
Atovaquone–proguanil combination tablet	One dose daily. 11–20 kg: 62.5 mg atovaquone plus 25 mg proguanil (1 paediatric tablet) daily 21–30 kg: 2 paediatric tablets daily 31–40 kg: 3 paediatric tablets daily > 40 kg: 1 adult tablet (250 mg atovaquone plus 100 mg proguanil) daily	Start 1 day before departure and continue for 7 days after return	No data, not recommended	No data, not recommended	Not recommended under 11 kg because of lack of data	Hypersensitivity to atovaquone and/or proguanil; severe renal insufficiency (creatinine clearance <30 ml/min).	Experience with this drug for prophylaxis in non-immune travellers is still limited. Plasma concentrations of atovaquone are reduced when it is co-administered with rifampicin, rifabutin, metoclopramide or tetracycline.
Choroquine	5 mg base/kg weekly, or 10 mg base/kg weekly divided in 6 daily doses adult dose: 300 mg chloroquine base weekly in one dose or 600 mg chloroquine base weekly divided over 6 daily doses of 100 mg base (with one drug-free day per week)	Start 1 week before departure and continue for 4 weeks after return	Safe	Safe	Safe	Hypersensitivity to chloroquine; history of epilepsy; psoriasis.	Concurrent use of chloroquine can reduce the antibody response to human diploid-cell rabies vaccine.
Chloroquine–proguanil combination tablet	> 50 kg: 100 mg chloroquine plus 200 mg proguanil (1 tablet) daily	Start 1 week before departure and continue for 4 weeks after return	Safe	Safe	Tablet size not suitable for persons of < 50 kg body weight	Hypersensitivity to chloroquine and/or proguanil; liver or kidney insufficiency; history of epilepsy; psoriasis.	Concurrent use of chloroquine can reduce the antibody response to human diploid-cell rabies vaccine.

Table 7.2 Use of antimalarial drugs for prophylaxis in travellers (*continued*)

Generic name	Dosage regimen	Duration of prophylaxis	Use in special groups			Contraindications	Comments
			Pregnancy	Breast-feeding	Children		
Doxycycline	1.5 mg salt/kg daily *adult dose:* 1 tablet of 100 mg daily	Start 1 day before departure and continue for 4 weeks after return.	Contra-indicated	Contra-indicated	Contra-indicated under 8 years of age	Hypersensitivity to tetra-cyclines; liver dysfunction.	Doxycycline makes the skin more susceptible to sunburn. People with sensitive skin should use a highly protective (UVA) sunscreen and avoid prolonged direct sunlight, or switch to another drug. Doxycycline should be taken with plenty of water to prevent oesophageal irritation. Doxycycline may increase the risk of vaginal *Candida* infections.
Mefloquine	5 mg/kg weekly *adult dose:* 1 tablet of 250 mg weekly	Start at least 1 week (preferably 2–3 weeks) before departure and continue for 4 weeks after return	Not recom-mended in first tri-mester because of lack of data	Safe	Not recom-mended under 5 kg because of lack of data	Hypersensitivity to mefloquine; psychiatric (including depres-sion) or convulsive disorders; history of severe neuropsychia-tric disease; concomitant halofantrine treatment; treat-ment with mefloquine in previous 4 weeks; people performing activities requiring fine coordination and spatial discrimination, e.g. pilots, machine operators.	Do not give mefloquine within 12 hours of quinine treatment. Mefloquine and other cardioactive drugs may be given concomitantly only under close medical supervision. Ampicillin, tetracycline and metoclopramide can increase mefloquine blood levels. Vaccination with live bacterial vaccines (e.g. oral live typhoid vaccine, cholera vaccine) should be completed at least 3 days before the first prophylactic dose of mefloquine.
Proguanil	3 mg/kg daily *adult dose:* 2 tablets of 100 mg daily	Start 1 day before departure and continue for 4 weeks after return	Safe	Safe	Safe	Liver or kidney dysfunction.	Use only in combination with chloroquine.

Table 7.3 **Use of antimalarial drugs for treatment of uncomplicated malaria in travellers**

Generic name	Dosage regimen	Use in special groups			Contraindications	Comments
		Pregnancy	Breast-feeding	Children		
Amodiaquine	30 mg base/kg taken in 3 daily doses	Apparently safe but limited data	Apparently safe but limited data	Safe	Hypersensitivity to amodiaquine; hepatic disorders.	
Artemether/ lumefantrine combination tablet	3-day course of 6 doses total, taken at 0, 8, 24, 36, 48, and 60 hours 10–14 kg: 1 tablet (20 mg artemether plus 120 mg lumefantrine) per dose 15–24 kg: 2 tablets per dose 25–34 kg: 3 tablets per dose 35 kg and over: 4 tablets per dose	No data, not recommended	No data, not recommended	Not recommended under 10 kg because of lack of data	Hypersensitivity to artemether and/or lumefantrine.	Experience with this drug for treatment of non-immune travellers is still limited. Better absorbed in the presence of fatty foods.
Artemisinin and derivatives	Artemisinin: 10 mg/kg daily for 7 days Artemisinin derivatives: 2 mg/kg daily for 7 days Artemisinin and its derivatives are given with a double divided dose on the first day	Not recommended in first trimester because of lack of data	Safe	Safe	Hypersensitivity to artemisinins.	As monotherapy these drugs should be taken for a minimum of 7 days, to prevent recrudescences. The duration of treatment may be reduced to 3 days when they are taken in combination with another effective antimalarial.
Atovaquone/ proguanil combination tablet	One dose daily for three consecutive days 11–20 kg: 1 adult tablet (250 mg atovaquone plus 100 mg proguanil) daily 21–30 kg: 2 adult tablets daily 31–40 kg: 3 adult tablets daily > 40 kg: 4 adult tablets (1 g atovaquone plus 400 mg proguanil) daily	No data, not recommended	No data, not recommended	Not recommended under 11 kg because of lack of data	Hypersensitivity to atovaquone and/or proguanil; severe renal insufficiency (creatinine clearance < 30 ml/min).	Experience with this drug for treatment of non-immune travellers is still limited. Plasma concentrations of atovaquone are reduced when the drug is co-administered with rifampicin, rifabutin, metoclopramide or tetracycline.
Chloroquine	25 mg base/kg divided in 3 daily doses (10, 10, 5 mg base/kg)	Safe	Safe	Safe	Hypersensitivity to chloroquine; history of epilepsy; psoriasis.	Concurrent use of chloroquine can reduce the antibody response to human diploid-cell rabies vaccine.

Table 7.3 Use of antimalarial drugs for treatment of uncomplicated malaria in travellers (continued)

Generic name	Dosage regimen	Use in special groups			Contraindications	Comments
		Pregnancy	Breast-feeding	Children		
Clindamycin	Under 60 kg: 5 mg base/kg 4 times daily for 5 days 60 kg and over: 300 mg base 4 times daily for 5 days	Apparently safe but limited data	Apparently safe but limited data	Apparently safe but limited data	Hypersensitivity to clindamycin or lincomycin; history of gastrointestinal disease, particularly colitis; severe liver or kidney impairment.	Used in combination with quinine in areas of emerging quinine resistance.
Doxycycline	Adults > 50 kg: 800 mg salt over 7 days, taken as 2 tablets (100 mg salt each) 12 hours apart on day 1, followed by 1 tablet daily for 6 days Children 8 years and older: 25–35 kg: 0.5 tablet per dose 36–50 kg: 0.75 tablet per dose > 50 kg: 1 tablet per dose	Contra-indicated	Contra-indicated	Contra-indicated under 8 years of age	Hypersensitivity to tetracyclines; liver dysfunction.	Used in combination with quinine in areas of emerging quinine resistance.
Halofantrine	8 mg base/kg in 3 doses at 6-hour intervals. Repeat full course after 1 week	No data, not recommended	No data, not recommended	Not recommended under 10 kg because of lack of data	Allergy to halofantrine; pre-existing cardiac disease; family history of sudden death or congenital prolongation of the QTc interval; use of other drugs or presence of a clinical condition known to prolong the QTc interval; treatment with mefloquine in the previous 3 weeks.	Risk of fatal cardiotoxicity. Only to be used in well-equipped medical facilities under close medical supervision.

Table 7.3 Use of antimalarial drugs for treatment of uncomplicated malaria in travellers (continued)

Generic name	Dosage regimen	Use in special groups			Contraindications	Comments
		Pregnancy	Breast-feeding	Children		
Mefloquine	15 mg base/kg as single dose, or 25 mg base/kg as split dose (15 mg/kg plus 10 mg/kg 6–24 hours apart) Mefloquine split dose (25 mg base/kg) in areas with resistance to mefloquine (e.g. Thai border areas)	Not recommended in first trimester because of lack of data	Safe	Not recommended under 5 kg because of lack of data	Hypersensitivity to mefloquine; psychiatric (including depression) or convulsive disorders; history of severe neuropsychiatric disease; concomitant halofantrine treatment; treatment with mefloquine in previous 4 weeks; people whose activities require fine coordination and spatial discrimination, e.g. pilots and machine operators.	Do not give mefloquine within 12 hours of last dose of quinine treatment. Mefloquine and other related compounds (such as quinine, quinidine, chloroquine) may be given concomitantly only under close medical supervision because of possible additive cardiac toxicity and increased risk of convulsions; co-administration of mefloquine with anti-arrhythmic agents, beta-adrenergic blocking agents, calcium channel blockers, antihistamines including H1-blocking agents, and phenothiazines may contribute to prolongation of QTc interval. Ampicillin, tetracycline and metoclopramide can increase mefloquine blood levels.
Primaquine	*Infections acquired south of the equator:* 0.5 mg base/kg for 14 days; *Infections acquired north of the equator:* 0.25 mg base/kg for 14 days	Contra-indicated	Safe	Contra-indicated under 4 years of age	G6PD deficiency; active rheumatoid arthritis; lupus erythematosus; conditions that predispose to granulocytopenia; concomitant use of drugs that may induce haematological disorders; concomitant use of quinine (reduces primaquine plasma levels).	Anti-relapse treatment of *P. vivax* and *P. ovale* infections.

Table 7.3 Use of antimalarial drugs for treatment of uncomplicated malaria in travellers *(continued)*

Generic name	Dosage regimen	Use in special groups			Contraindications	Comments
		Pregnancy	Breast-feeding	Children		
Quinine	8 mg base/kg 3 times daily for 7 days	Safe	Safe	Safe	Hypersensitivity to quinine or quinidine; tinnitus; optic neuritis; haemolysis; myasthenia gravis. Use with caution in persons with G6PD deficiency, and in patients with atrial fibrillation, cadiac conduction defects, or heart block. Quinine may enhance effect of cardiosuppressant drugs. Use with caution in persons using beta blockers, digoxin, calcium channel blockers, etc.	In areas of high-level resistance to quinine: give in combination with doxycycline, tetracycline or clindamycin. Quinine may induce hypoglycaemia, particularly in (malnourished) children, pregnant women and patients with severe disease.
Sulfadoxine–pyrimethamine combination tablet	5–60 kg: single dose calculated as 25mg/kg of the sulfa component 60 kg and over: single dose of 3 tablets (1500 mg sulfadoxine plus 75 mg pyrimethamine)	Safe with caution at term	Safe with caution	Contraindicated under 2 months of age	Hypersensitivity to sulfa drugs or pyrimethamine; severe liver or kidney dysfunction; megaloblastic anaemia; concomitant use of other sulfa drugs or folate antagonists.	Cutaneous drug reactions more common in people infected with HIV.
Tetracycline	25–49 kg: 5 mg salt/kg 4 times daily for 7 days 50 kg and over: 250 mg salt (1 tablet) 4 times daily for 7 days	Contra-indicated	Contra-indicated	Contra-indicated under 8 years of age	Hypersensitivity to tetracyclines; liver or kidney dysfunction; systemic lupus erythematosus; caution in patients with myasthenia gravis.	Used in combination with quinine in areas of emerging quinine resistance.

Countries and territories with malarious areas

The following list shows all countries where malaria occurs. In some of these countries, malaria is present only in certain areas or up to a particular altitude. In many countries, malaria has a seasonal pattern. These details are provided in the country list, together with information on the predominant malaria species, status of resistance to antimalarial drugs and recommended chemoprophylactic regimen.

(* *P. vivax* risk only)

Afghanistan
Algeria*
Angola
Argentina*
Armenia*
Azerbaijan*
Bangladesh
Belize
Benin
Bhutan
Bolivia
Botswana
Brazil
Burkina Faso
Burundi
Cambodia
Cameroon
Cape Verde
Central African Republic
Chad
China
Colombia
Comoros
Congo
Congo, Democratic
   Republic of the
   (former Zaire)
Costa Rica
Côte d'Ivoire
Djibouti
Dominican Republic
East Timor
Ecuador
Egypt
El Salvador
Equatorial Guinea
Eritrea

Ethiopia
French Guiana
Gabon
Gambia
Georgia*
Ghana
Guatemala
Guinea
Guinea-Bissau
Guyana
Haiti
Honduras
India
Indonesia
Iran, Islamic Republic of
Iraq*
Kenya
Korea, Democratic
   People's Republic of*
Korea, Republic of*
Lao People's Democratic
   Republic
Liberia
Madagascar
Malawi
Malaysia
Mali
Mauritania
Mauritius*
Mayotte
Mexico
Morocco*
Mozambique
Myanmar
Namibia
Nepal
Nicaragua

Niger
Nigeria
Oman
Pakistan
Panama
Papua New Guinea
Paraguay
Peru
Philippines
Rwanda
Sao Tome and Principe
Saudi Arabia
Senegal
Sierra Leone
Solomon Islands
Somalia
South Africa
Sri Lanka
Sudan
Suriname
Swaziland
Syrian Arab Republic*
Tajikistan
Tanzania, United
   Republic of
Thailand
Togo
Turkey*
Turkmenistan*
Uganda
United Arab Emirates
Vanuatu
Venezuela
Viet Nam
Yemen
Zambia
Zimbabwe

CHAPTER 8
Blood transfusion

Blood transfusion is a life-saving intervention provided that it is carried out correctly and that the transfused blood is safe for the recipient. Because of inherent risks, transfusion should be prescribed only for conditions for which there is no other treatment.

For travellers, the need for a blood transfusion is almost always due to a medical emergency involving sudden massive blood loss, such as:

— traffic accident
— gynaecological and obstetric emergencies
— severe gastrointestinal haemorrhage
— emergency surgery.

The safety of blood and blood products depends on careful selection of donors, testing all donations for transfusion-transmissible infectious agents and rigorous control of all procedures involved in donation, testing and transfusion.

The safety of transfusion depends on appropriate prescription (only when there is no other remedy), careful checking of compatibility of the blood or blood product with the recipient's blood, and rigorous control of all procedures involved.

In many developing countries, safe blood products and the expertise to prescribe and carry out safe transfusion are not available in health care facilities. The risks associated with unsafe blood transfusion are:

— incompatibility of transfused blood owing to failure to carry out careful compatibility testing;
— transfusion of infectious agents that cause diseases such as HIV, malaria, hepatitis B, hepatitis C, syphilis, Chagas disease (as a result of their presence in the transfused blood or on transfusion equipment).

Initial management to prevent further blood loss by positioning the patient correctly helps to maintain adequate blood pressure and flow of blood to vital organs.

In many cases, transfusion of blood can be avoided by replacing the blood volume with plasma substitutes (crystalloids or colloids). In areas where malaria occurs, transfused patients should receive antimalaria therapy as a routine precaution.

Precautions

- Travellers should carry a medical card or other document, showing their blood group and information about any current medical problems or treatment.

- Unnecessary travel should be avoided by those with pre-existing conditions that may give rise to a need for blood transfusion.

- Travellers should take all possible precautions to avoid involvement in traffic accidents (see Chapter 4).

- Travellers may obtain in advance a contact address at the travel destination for advice and assistance in case of medical emergency.

- Travellers with medical conditions such as haemophilia, who may need blood transfusion, must take medical advice in advance and identify appropriate medical facilities at the travel destination.

- Travellers with a medical condition that necessitates transfusion of plasma-derived products to replace coagulation factor or immunoglobulin should obtain medical advice and make appropriate arrangements in advance.

Further reading

The clinical use of blood: handbook. Geneva, WHO, 2001.

Country list
Vaccination requirements and malaria situation[1]

Introduction

The information provided for each country includes the name and approximate altitude of the capital city, the requirements for mandatory yellow fever vaccination where these apply, and details concerning the malaria situation and recommended prophylaxis.

Yellow fever vaccination

Yellow fever vaccination is carried out for two different purposes:

- *To protect individual travellers* who may be exposed to yellow fever infection. Vaccination in these cases is recommended but not mandatory. As yellow fever is frequently fatal for those who have not been vaccinated, vaccination is recommended for all travellers (with few exceptions—see Chapter 6) intending to visit areas where there may be a risk of exposure to yellow fever.
- *To protect countries* from the risk of importing yellow fever virus. This is mandatory vaccination and is a requirement for entry into the countries concerned.

Travellers should be warned that the requirement for vaccination against yellow fever is not related to the risk of exposure to the disease.

The countries that require proof of vaccination[2] are those where the disease does *not* occur but where the mosquito vector and non-human primate hosts of yellow fever are present. Consequently, any importation of the virus by an infected traveller could result in its establishment and propagation in the local mosquitoes and primates, leading to a risk of infection for the human population.

---

[1] For the purpose of this publication, the term "country" covers countries, territories and areas.

[2] Please note that the requirements for vaccination of infants over 6 months of age by some countries is not in accordance with WHO's recommendations (see Chapter 6). Travellers should however be informed that the requirement exists for entry into the countries concerned.

Proof of vaccination is required for all travellers coming *from* countries where yellow fever occurs, including transit through such countries. The international yellow fever vaccination certificate becomes valid 10 days after vaccination and remains valid for a period of 10 years.

The fact that a country has no mandatory requirement for vaccination does *not* imply that there is no risk of yellow fever infection.

In accordance with the International Health Regulations, countries are required to notify all cases of yellow fever to WHO. Such countries are then considered to be "infected areas". This terminology is likely to change in the revised version of the Regulations, but is meantime retained in the following country list to maintain consistency with the official reports provided by the WHO Member States. The list of infected areas is published in the *Weekly epidemiological record*.

In addition, countries are considered to be "endemic areas" for yellow fever if the virus is present in mosquitoes and non-human primates and where there is therefore a potential risk of infection for humans (see map, page 84).

Other

Routine vaccination (see Chapter 6). It is recommended that all travellers are fully vaccinated with the appropriate routine vaccines; schedules for booster doses should be followed at the recommended time intervals.

Cholera. No country requires a certificate of vaccination against cholera as a condition for entry. For information on selective use of cholera vaccines, see Chapter 6.

Smallpox. Since the global eradication of smallpox was certified in 1980, WHO does not recommend smallpox vaccination for travellers.

Hepatitis A. Vaccination against hepatitis A is recommended for all travellers to developing countries and to countries with economies in transition.

Information on other vaccines for selective use is given in Chapter 6.

Infectious diseases. Information on the main infectious disease threats for travellers, their geographical distribution, and corresponding precautions is provided in Chapter 5.

Malaria. General information about the disease, its geographical distribution and details of preventive measures are included in Chapter 7. Specific information for each country is provided in this section, including epidemiological details for all countries with malarious areas (geographical and seasonal distribution, altitude, predominant species, status of resistance). The recommended chemoprophylactic regimen is also indicated. The recommended prophylaxis for each country is decided on the basis of the following factors: the risk of contracting malaria; the prevailing species of malaria parasites in the area; the level and spread of drug resistance reported from the country; and the possible risk of serious side-effects resulting from the use of the various prophylactic drugs.

The following abbreviations are used: CHL = chloroquine; C+P = chloroquine plus proguanil; MEF = mefloquine; DOX = doxycycline.

Please note that altitudes quoted in this list are averages for guidance only.

AFGHANISTAN

Capital Kabul

Altitude 1800 m

Yellow fever: A yellow fever vaccination certificate is required from travellers coming from infected areas.

Malaria: Malaria risk—*P. vivax* and *P. falciparum*—exists from May through November below 2000 m. Chloroquine-resistant *P. falciparum* reported.

Recommended prophylaxis: C+P.

ALBANIA

Capital Tirana

Altitude 130 m

Yellow fever: A yellow fever vaccination certificate is required from travellers over 1 year of age coming from infected areas.

ALGERIA

Capital Algiers

Altitude 30 m

Yellow fever: A yellow fever vaccination certificate is required from travellers over 1 year of age coming from infected areas.

Malaria: Malaria risk is limited. One small focus (*P. vivax*) has been reported in Ihrir (Illizi Department), but this is isolated and access is difficult.

Recommended prophylaxis: none.

AMERICAN SAMOA

Capital Pago Pago

Altitude 10 m

Yellow fever: A yellow fever vaccination certificate is required from travellers over 1 year of age coming from infected areas.

ANDORRA

Capital Andorra la Vella

Altitude 1410 m

No vaccination requirements for any international traveller.

ANGOLA

Capital Luanda

Altitude 10 m

Yellow fever: A yellow fever vaccination certificate is required from travellers over 1 year of age coming from infected areas.

Malaria: Malaria risk—predominantly due to *P. falciparum*—exists throughout the year in the whole country. *P. falciparum* resistant to chloroquine and sulfadoxine–pyrimethamine reported.

Recommended prophylaxis: MEF.

ANGUILLA

Capital The Valley

Altitude 0 m

Yellow fever: A yellow fever vaccination certificate is required from travellers over 1 year of age coming from infected areas.

ANTIGUA AND BARBUDA

Capital St John's

Altitude 0 m

Yellow fever: A yellow fever vaccination certificate is required from travellers over 1 year of age coming from infected areas.

ARGENTINA

Capital Buenos Aires

Altitude 30 m

No vaccination requirements for any international traveller.

Malaria: Malaria risk—exclusively due to *P. vivax* —is low and is confined to rural areas along the borders with Bolivia (lowlands of Jujuy and Salta provinces) and with Paraguay (lowlands of Corrientes and Misiones provinces).

Recommended prophylaxis in risk areas: CHL.

ARMENIA

Capital Yerevan
Altitude 1000 m
No vaccination requirements for any international traveller.

Malaria: Malaria risk—exclusively due to *P. vivax*—exists focally from June through October in some of the villages located in Ararat Valley, mainly in the Masis district. No risk in tourist areas.

Recommended prophylaxis: none.

AUSTRALIA

Capital Canberra
Altitude 610 m
Yellow fever: A yellow fever vaccination certificate is required from travellers over 1 year of age entering Australia within 6 days of having stayed overnight or longer in an infected country, as listed in the *Weekly epidemiological record*.

AUSTRIA

Capital Vienna
Altitude 170 m
No vaccination requirements for any international traveller.

AZERBAIJAN

Capital Baku
Altitude 0 m
No vaccination requirements for any international traveller.

Malaria: Limited malaria risk—exclusively due to *P. vivax*—exists from June through September in lowland areas, mainly in the area between the Kura and the Arax rivers.

Recommended prophylaxis: none.

BAHAMAS

Capital Nassau
Altitude 10 m
Yellow fever: A yellow fever vaccination certificate is required from travellers over 1 year of age coming from infected areas.

BAHRAIN

Capital Manama
Altitude 0 m
No vaccination requirements for any international traveller.

BANGLADESH

Capital Dhaka
Altitude 10 m
Yellow fever: Any person (including infants) who arrives by air or sea without a certificate is detained in isolation for a period of up to 6 days if arriving within 6 days of departure from an infected area or having been in transit in such an area, or having come by an aircraft that has been in an infected area and has not been disinsected in accordance with the procedure and formulation laid down in Schedule VI of the Bangladesh Aircraft (Public Health) Rules 1977 (First Amendment) or those recommended by WHO.

The following countries and areas are regarded as infected:

Africa: Angola, Benin, Burkina Faso, Burundi, Cameroon, Central African Republic, Chad, Congo, Côte d'Ivoire, Democratic Republic of the Congo, Equatorial Guinea, Ethiopia, Gabon, Gambia, Ghana, Guinea, Guinea-Bissau, Kenya, Liberia, Malawi, Mali, Mauritania, Niger, Nigeria, Rwanda, Sao Tome and Principe, Senegal, Sierra Leone, Somalia, Sudan (south of 15°N), Togo, Uganda, United Republic of Tanzania, Zambia.

America: Belize, Bolivia, Brazil, Colombia, Costa Rica, Ecuador, French Guiana, Guatemala, Guyana, Honduras, Nicaragua, Panama, Peru, Suriname, Trinidad and Tobago, Venezuela.

Note. When a case of yellow fever is reported from any country, that country is regarded by the Government of Bangladesh as infected with yellow fever and is added to the above list.

Malaria: Malaria risk exists throughout the year in the whole country, excluding Dhaka city. *P. falciparum* resistant to chloroquine reported in the south-east; resistance to sulfadoxine– pyrimethamine also reported.

Recommended prophylaxis: C+P; in forested areas and south-east, MEF.

BARBADOS

Capital Bridgetown
Altitude 10 m
Yellow fever: A yellow fever vaccination certificate is required from travellers over 1 year of age coming from infected areas.

BELARUS

Capital Minsk
Altitude 210 m
No vaccination requirements for any international traveller

BELGIUM

Capital Brussels
Altitude 80 m
No vaccination requirements for any international traveller

BELIZE

Capital Belmopan
Altitude 60 m
Yellow fever: A yellow fever vaccination certificate is required from travellers coming from infected areas.

Malaria: Malaria risk—almost exclusively due to *P. vivax*—exists in all districts but varies within regions. Risk is highest in the western and southern regions. No resistant *P. falciparum* strains reported.

Recommended prophylaxis in risk areas: CHL.

BENIN

Capital Porto-Novo (constitutional) /
Cotonou (seat of Government)
Altitude 40 m / 50 m
Yellow fever: A yellow fever vaccination certificate is required from all travellers over 1 year of age.

Malaria: Malaria risk—predominantly due to *P. falciparum*—exists throughout the year in the whole country. Chloroquine-resistant *P. falciparum* reported.

Recommended prophylaxis: MEF.

BERMUDA

Capital Hamilton
Altitude 0 m
No vaccination requirements for any international traveller.

BHUTAN

Capital Thimphu
Altitude 2740 m
Yellow fever: A yellow fever vaccination certificate is required from travellers coming from infected areas.

Malaria: Malaria risk exists throughout the year in the southern belt of five districts: Chirang, Samchi, Samdrupjongkhar, Sarpang and Shemgang. *P. falciparum* resistant to chloroquine and sulfadoxine–pyrimethamine reported.

Recommended prophylaxis in risk areas: C+P.

BOLIVIA

Capital La Paz (administrative) /
Sucre (legislative)
Altitude 3700 m / 2800 m
Yellow fever: A yellow fever vaccination certificate is required from travellers coming from infected areas. Vaccination is recommended for incoming travellers from non-infected zones visiting risk areas such as the departments of Beni, Cochabamba and Santa Cruz, and the subtropical part of La Paz Department.

Malaria: Malaria risk—predominantly due to *P. vivax*—exists throughout the year below 2500 m in the departments of Beni, Pando, Santa Cruz and Tarija, and in the provinces of Lacareja, Rurenabaque, and North and South Yungas in La Paz Department. Lower risk exists in Cochabamba and Chuquisaca. Falciparum malaria occurs in Beni and Pando, especially in the localities of Guayaramerín, Puerto Rico and Riberalta. *P. falciparum* resistant to chloroquine and sulfadoxine–pyrimethamine reported.

Recommended prophylaxis in risk areas: CHL; in northern departments, MEF.

BOSNIA AND HERZEGOVINA

Capital Sarajevo
Altitude 520 m
No vaccination requirements for any international traveller.

BOTSWANA

Capital Gaborone
Altitude 1000 m
No vaccination requirements for any international traveller.

Malaria: Malaria risk—predominantly due to *P. falciparum*—exists from November to May/June in the northern parts of the country: Boteti, Chobe, Ngamiland, Okavango, Tutume districts/sub-districts. Chloroquine-resistant *P. falciparum* reported.

Recommended prophylaxis in risk areas: MEF.

BRAZIL

Capital Brasilia

Altitude 1000 m

Yellow fever: A yellow fever vaccination certificate is required from travellers over 9 months of age coming from infected areas, unless they are in possession of a waiver stating that immunization is contraindicated on medical grounds. The following countries or areas are regarded as infected:

Africa: Angola, Cameroon, Democratic Republic of the Congo, Gabon, Gambia, Ghana, Guinea, Liberia, Nigeria, Sierra Leone, Sudan.

America: Bolivia, Colombia, Ecuador, Peru.

Vaccination is recommended for travellers to endemic areas, including rural areas in the states of Acre, Amapá, Amazonas, Goiás, Maranhão, Mato Grosso, Mato Grosso do Sul, Pará, Rondônia, Roraima and Tocantins, and certain areas of Minas Gerais, Parana and São Paulo.

Malaria: Malaria risk—*P. vivax* (78%), *P. falciparum* (22%)—is high throughout the year in most forested areas below 900 m within the nine states of the "Legal Amazonia" region (Acre, Amapá, Amazonas, Maranhão (western part), Mato Grosso (northern part), Pará (except Belém City), Rondônia, Roraima and Tocantins. Transmission intensity varies from municipality to municipality, but is very high in jungle areas of mining, lumbering and agricultural settlements less than 5 years old where multidrug-resistant *P. falciparum* strains are common (> 50%). Intensity of transmission is lower in urban areas, including in large cities such as Pôrto Velho, Boa Vista, Macapá, Manaus, Santarém and Maraba. In the states outside "Legal Amazonia", malaria transmission risk is negligible or non-existent.

Recommended prophylaxis in risk areas: MEF.

BRITISH VIRGIN ISLANDS

Capital Road Town

Altitude 0 m

No vaccination requirements for any international traveller.

BRUNEI DARUSSALAM

Capital Bandar Seri Begawan

Altitude 0 m

Yellow fever: A yellow fever vaccination certificate is required from travellers over 1 year of age coming from infected areas or having passed through partly or wholly endemic areas within the preceding 6 days. The countries and areas included in the endemic zones are considered as infected areas.

BULGARIA

Capital Sofia

Altitude 570 m

No vaccination requirements for any international traveller.

BURKINA FASO

Capital Ouagadougou

Altitude 320 m

Yellow fever: A yellow fever vaccination certificate is required from all travellers over 1 year of age.

Malaria: Malaria risk—predominantly due to *P. falciparum*—exists throughout the year in the whole country. Resistance to chloroquine reported.

Recommended prophylaxis: MEF.

BURMA *see* MYANMAR

BURUNDI

Capital Bujumbura

Altitude 780 m

Yellow fever: A yellow fever vaccination certificate is required from travellers over 1 year of age coming from infected areas.

Malaria: Malaria risk—predominantly due to *P. falciparum*—exists throughout the year in the whole country. Resistance to chloroquine reported.

Recommended prophylaxis: MEF.

CAMBODIA

Capital Phnom Penh

Altitude 20 m

Yellow fever: A yellow fever vaccination certificate is required from travellers coming from infected areas.

Malaria: Malaria risk—predominantly due to *P. falciparum*—exists throughout the year in the whole country except in the Phnom Penh area and close around Tonle Sap. Malaria does, however, occur in the tourist area of Angkor Wat. *P. falciparum* resistant to chloroquine and sulfadoxine–pyrimethamine reported. Resistance to mefloquine reported in western provinces near the Thai border.

Recommended prophylaxis (including Battambang and Angkor Wat areas): MEF; in western provinces, DOX.

CAMEROON

Capital Yaoundé
Altitude 730 m
Yellow fever: A yellow fever vaccination certificate is required from all travellers over 1 year of age.

Malaria: Malaria risk—predominantly due to *P. falciparum*—exists throughout the year in the whole country. *P. falciparum* resistant to chloroquine and sulfadoxine–pyrimethamine reported.

Recommended prophylaxis: MEF.

CANADA

Capital Ottawa
Altitude 80 m
No vaccination requirements for any international traveller.

CAPE VERDE

Capital Praia
Altitude 0 m
Yellow fever: A yellow fever vaccination certificate is required from travellers over 1 year of age coming from countries having notified cases in the last 6 years.

Malaria: Limited malaria risk exists from September through November in São Tiago Island.

Recommended prophylaxis: none.

CAYMAN ISLANDS

Capital Georgetown
Altitude 0 m
No vaccination requirements for any international traveller

CENTRAL AFRICAN REPUBLIC

Capital Bangui
Altitude 380 m
Yellow fever: A yellow fever vaccination certificate is required from all travellers over 1 year of age.

Malaria: Malaria risk—predominantly due to *P. falciparum*—exists throughout the year in the whole country. Resistance to chloroquine and sulfadoxine–pyrimethamine reported.

Recommended prophylaxis: MEF.

CHAD

Capital N'Djamena
Altitude 300 m
Yellow fever: Yellow fever vaccination is recommended for all travellers over 1 year of age.

Malaria: Malaria risk—predominantly due to *P. falciparum*—exists throughout the year in the whole country. Resistance to chloroquine reported.

Recommended prophylaxis: MEF.

CHILE

Capital Santiago
Altitude 520 m
No vaccination requirements for any international traveller.

CHINA

Capital Beijing
Altitude 60 m
Yellow fever: A yellow fever vaccination certificate is required from travellers coming from infected areas.

Malaria: Malaria risk—including *P. falciparum* malaria—occurs in Hainan and Yunnan. Multidrug-resistant *P. falciparum* has been reported. Risk of *P. vivax* malaria exists in Fujian, Guangdong, Guangxi, Guizhou, Hainan, Sichuan, Xizang (only along the valley of the Zangbo river in the extreme south-east) and Yunnan. Very low malaria risk (*P. vivax* only) exists in Anhui, Hubei, Hunan, Jiangsu, Jiangxi and Shandong. The risk may be higher in areas of focal outbreaks. Where transmission exists, it occurs only in remote rural communities below 1500 m: from July to November north of latitude 33°N, from May to December between 33°N and 25°N, and throughout the year south of 25°N. There is no malaria risk in urban areas nor in the densely populated plain areas. In general, tourists do not need to take malaria prophylaxis unless they plan to stay in remote rural areas in the provinces listed above.

Recommended prophylaxis in risk areas: CHL; in Hainan and Yunnan, MEF.

CHINA, HONG KONG SAR

Capital Hong Kong
Altitude 30 m
No vaccination requirements for any international traveller.

CHINA, MACAO SAR

Capital Macao
Altitude 10 m
No vaccination requirements for any international traveller.

CHRISTMAS ISLAND

(Indian Ocean)

Capital The Settlement
Altitude 0 m
Same requirements as mainland Australia.

COLOMBIA

Capital Bogotá
Altitude 2600 m
Yellow fever: Vaccination is recommended for travellers who may visit the following areas considered to be endemic for yellow fever: middle valley of the Magdalena river, eastern and western foothills of the Cordillera Oriental from the frontier with Ecuador to that with Venezuela, Urabá, foothills of the Sierra Nevada, eastern plains (Orinoquia) and Amazonia.

Malaria: Malaria risk—*P. falciparum* (37%), *P. vivax* (63%)—is high throughout the year in rural/jungle areas below 800 m, especially in municipalities of the regions of Amazonia, Orinoquía, Pacífico and Urabá-Bajo Cauca. Transmission intensity varies from department to department, with the highest risk in Amazonas, Chocó, Córdoba, Guainía, Guaviare, Putumayo and Vichada. Chloroquine-resistant *P. falciparum* exists in Amazonia, Pacífico and Urabá-Bajo Cauca. Resistance to sulfadoxine–pyrimethamine reported.

Recommended prophylaxis in risk areas: C+P; in Amazonia, Pacífico and Urabá-Bajo Cauca, MEF.

COMOROS

Capital Moroni
Altitude 10 m
No vaccination requirements for any international traveller.

Malaria: Malaria risk—predominantly due to *P. falciparum*—exists throughout the year in the whole country. Resistance to chloroquine reported.

Recommended prophylaxis: MEF.

CONGO

Capital Brazzaville
Altitude 300 m
Yellow fever: A yellow fever vaccination certificate is required from all travellers over 1 year of age.

Malaria: Malaria risk—predominantly due to *P. falciparum*—exists throughout the year in the whole country. Resistance to chloroquine reported.

Recommended prophylaxis: MEF.

CONGO, DEMOCRATIC REPUBLIC OF THE (formerly ZAIRE)

Capital Kinshasa
Altitude 200 m
Yellow fever: A yellow fever vaccination certificate is required from travellers over 1 year of age.

Malaria: Malaria risk—predominantly due to *P. falciparum*—exists throughout the year in the whole country. Resistance to chloroquine and sulfadoxine–pyrimethamine reported.

Recommended prophylaxis: MEF.

COOK ISLANDS

Capital Avarua
Altitude 210 m
No vaccination requirements for any international traveller.

COSTA RICA

Capital San José
Altitude 1160 m

No vaccination requirements for any international traveller.

Malaria: Malaria risk—almost exclusively due to *P. vivax*—is moderate throughout the year in the cantons of Los Chiles (Alajuela Province) and Matina and Talamanca (Limón Province). Lower transmission risk exists in cantons in the provinces of Alajuela, Guanacaste and Heredia, and in other cantons in Limón Province. Negligible or no risk of malaria transmission exists in the other cantons of the country.

Recommended prophylaxis in risk areas: CHL.

CÔTE D'IVOIRE

Capital Yamoussoukro / Abidjan (seat of Government)

Altitude 220 m / 50 m

Yellow fever: A yellow fever vaccination certificate is required from all travellers over 1 year of age.

Malaria: Malaria risk—predominantly due to *P. falciparum*—exists throughout the year in the whole country. Resistance to chloroquine and sulfadoxine–pyrimethamine reported.

Recommended prophylaxis: MEF.

CROATIA

Capital Zagreb

Altitude 140 m

No vaccination requirements for any international traveller.

CUBA

Capital Havana

Altitude 30 m

No vaccination requirements for any international traveller.

CYPRUS

Capital Nicosia

Altitude 140 m

No vaccination requirements for any international traveller.

CZECH REPUBLIC

Capital Prague

Altitude 250 m

No vaccination requirements for any international traveller.

DENMARK

Capital Copenhagen

Altitude 0 m

No vaccination requirements for any international traveller.

DJIBOUTI

Capital Djibouti

Altitude 0 m

Yellow fever: A yellow fever vaccination certificate is required from travellers over 1 year of age coming from infected areas.

Malaria: Malaria risk—predominantly due to *P. falciparum*—exists throughout the year in the whole country. Chloroquine-resistant *P. falciparum* reported.

Recommended prophylaxis: MEF.

DOMINICA

Capital Roseau

Altitude 0 m

Yellow fever: A yellow fever vaccination certificate is required from travellers over 1 year of age coming from infected areas.

DOMINICAN REPUBLIC

Capital Santo Domingo

Altitude 380 m

No vaccination requirements for any international traveller.

Malaria: Low malaria risk—exclusively due to *P. falciparum*—exists throughout the year, especially in rural areas of the western provinces such as Castañuelas, Hondo Valle and Pepillo Salcedo. There is no evidence of *P. falciparum* resistance to any antimalarial drug.

Recommended prophylaxis in risk areas: CHL.

EAST TIMOR

Capital Dili

Altitude 0 m

No vaccination requirements for any international traveller.

Malaria: Malaria risk—predominantly due to *P. falciparum*—exists throughout the year in the whole territory. *P. falciparum* resistant to chloroquine and sulfadoxine–pyrimethamine reported.

Recommended prophylaxis: MEF or DOX.

ECUADOR

Capital Quito

Altitude 2800 m

Yellow fever: A yellow fever vaccination certificate is required from travellers over 1 year of age coming from infected areas.

Malaria: Malaria risk—*P. falciparum* (57%), *P. vivax* (43%)—exists throughout the year below 1500 m, with some risk in Cotopaxi, Loja and Los Rios. Higher transmission risk is found in El Oro, Esmeraldas and Manabi. There is no risk in Guayaquil or Quito. A high proportion of *P. falciparum* cases in Esmeraldas Province are reportedly resistant to chloroquine.

Recommended prophylaxis in risk areas: CHL; in Esmeraldas province, MEF.

EGYPT

Capital Cairo

Altitude 20 m

Yellow fever: A yellow fever vaccination certificate is required from travellers over 1 year of age coming from infected areas. The following countries and areas are regarded as infected areas; air passengers in transit coming from these countries or areas without a certificate will be detained in the precincts of the airport until they resume their journey:

Africa: Angola, Benin, Burkina Faso, Burundi, Cameroon, Central African Republic, Chad, Congo, Côte d'Ivoire, Democratic Republic of the Congo, Equatorial Guinea, Ethiopia, Gabon, Gambia, Ghana, Guinea, Guinea-Bissau, Kenya, Liberia, Mali, Niger, Nigeria, Rwanda, Sao Tome and Principe, Senegal, Sierra Leone, Somalia, Sudan (south of 15°N), Togo, Uganda, United Republic of Tanzania, Zambia.

America: Belize, Bolivia, Brazil, Colombia, Costa Rica, Ecuador, French Guiana, Guyana, Panama, Peru, Suriname, Trinidad and Tobago, Venezuela.

All arrivals from Sudan are required to possess either a vaccination certificate or a location certificate issued by a Sudanese official centre stating that they have not been in Sudan south of 15°N within the previous 6 days.

Malaria: Very limited *P. falciparum* and *P. vivax* malaria risk exists from June through October in El Faiyûm governorate (no cases reported since 1998).

Recommended prophylaxis: none.

EL SALVADOR

Capital San Salvador

Altitude 680 m

Yellow fever: A yellow fever vaccination certificate is required from travellers over 6 months of age coming from infected areas.

Malaria: Very low malaria risk—almost exclusively due to *P. vivax*—exists throughout the year in Santa Ana Province, in rural areas of migratory influence from Guatemala.

Recommended prophylaxis in risk areas: CHL.

EQUATORIAL GUINEA

Capital Malabo

Altitude 380 m

Yellow fever: A yellow fever vaccination certificate is required from travellers coming from infected areas.

Malaria: Malaria risk—predominantly due to *P. falciparum*—exists throughout the year in the whole country. Resistance to chloroquine and sulfadoxine–pyrimethamine reported.

Recommended prophylaxis: MEF.

ERITREA

Capital Asmara

Altitude 2400 m

Yellow fever: A yellow fever vaccination certificate is required from travellers coming from infected areas.

Malaria: Malaria risk—predominantly due to *P. falciparum*—exists throughout the year in the whole country below 2200 m. There is no risk in Asmara. Chloroquine-resistant *P. falciparum* reported.

Recommended prophylaxis: MEF.

ESTONIA

Capital Tallinn

Altitude 40 m

No vaccination requirements for any international traveller.

ETHIOPIA

Capital Addis Ababa

Altitude 2400 m

Yellow fever: A yellow fever vaccination certificate is required from travellers over 1 year of age coming from infected areas.

Malaria: Malaria risk—predominantly due to *P. falciparum*—exists throughout the year in the whole country below 2000 m. Chloroquine-resistant *P. falciparum* reported. There is no malaria risk in Addis Ababa.

Recommended prophylaxis: MEF.

FALKLAND ISLANDS (MALVINAS)

Capital Stanley

Altitude 0 m

No vaccination requirements for any international traveller.

FAROE ISLANDS

Capital Torshavn

Altitude 0 m

No vaccination requirements for any international traveller.

FIJI

Capital Suva

Altitude 10 m

Yellow fever: A yellow fever vaccination certificate is required from travellers over 1 year of age entering Fiji within 10 days of having stayed overnight or longer in infected areas.

FINLAND

Capital Helsinki

Altitude 20 m

No vaccination requirements for any international traveller.

FRANCE

Capital Paris

Altitude 40 m

No vaccination requirements for any international traveller.

FRENCH GUIANA

Capital Cayenne

Altitude 0 m

Yellow fever: A yellow fever vaccination certificate is required from all travellers over 1 year of age.

Malaria: Malaria risk—*P. falciparum* (89%), *P. vivax* (11%)—is high throughout the year in nine municipalities of the territory bordering Brazil (Oiapoque river valley) and Suriname (Maroni river valley). In the other 13 municipalities transmission risk is low or negligible. Multidrug-resistant *P. falciparum* reported in areas influenced by Brazilian migration.

Recommended prophylaxis in risk areas: MEF.

FRENCH POLYNESIA

Capital Papeete

Altitude 0 m

Yellow fever: A yellow fever vaccination certificate is required from travellers over 1 year of age coming from infected areas.

GABON

Capital Libreville

Altitude 10 m

Yellow fever: A yellow fever vaccination certificate is required from all travellers over 1 year of age.

Malaria: Malaria risk—predominantly due to *P. falciparum*—exists throughout the year in the whole country. Resistance to chloroquine and sulfadoxine–pyrimethamine reported.

Recommended prophylaxis: MEF.

GAMBIA

Capital Banjul

Altitude 0 m

Yellow fever: A yellow fever vaccination certificate is required from travellers over 1 year of age arriving from endemic or infected areas.

Malaria: Malaria risk—predominantly due to *P. falciparum*—exists throughout the year in the whole country. Resistance to chloroquine and sulfadoxine–pyrimethamine reported.

Recommended prophylaxis: MEF.

GEORGIA

Capital Tbilisi

Altitude 400 m

No vaccination requirements for any international traveller.

Malaria: Malaria risk—exclusively due to *P. vivax*—exists focally from July to October in some villages located in the south-eastern part of the country.

Recommended prophylaxis: none.

GERMANY

Capital Berlin
Altitude 50 m
No vaccination requirements for any international traveller.

GHANA

Capital Accra
Altitude 70 m
Yellow fever: A yellow fever vaccination certificate is required from all travellers.

Malaria: Malaria risk—predominantly due to *P. falciparum*—exists throughout the year in the whole country. Resistance to chloroquine and sulfadoxine–pyrimethamine reported.

Recommended prophylaxis: MEF.

GIBRALTAR

Capital Gibraltar
Altitude 450 m
No vaccination requirements for any international traveller.

GREECE

Capital Athens
Altitude 150 m
Yellow fever: A yellow fever vaccination certificate is required from travellers over 6 months of age coming from infected areas.

GREENLAND

Capital Nuuk
Altitude 0 m
No vaccination requirements for any international traveller.

GRENADA

Capital Saint George's
Altitude 30 m
Yellow fever: A yellow fever vaccination certificate is required from travellers over 1 year of age coming from infected areas.

GUADELOUPE

Capital Basse-Terre
Altitude 0 m
Yellow fever: A yellow fever vaccination certificate is required from travellers over 1 year of age coming from infected areas.

GUAM

Capital Agana
Altitude 0 m
No vaccination requirements for any international traveller.

GUATEMALA

Capital Guatemala City
Altitude 1500 m
Yellow fever: A yellow fever vaccination certificate is required from travellers over 1 year of age coming from countries with infected areas.

Malaria: Malaria risk—predominantly due to *P. vivax*—exists throughout the year below 1500 m. There is high risk in the departments of Alta Verapaz, Baja Verapaz, Petén and San Marcos, and moderate risk in the departments of Escuintla, Huehuetenango, Izabal, Quiché, Retalhuleu, Suchitepéquez and Zacapa.

Recommended prophylaxis in risk areas: CHL.

GUINEA

Capital Conakry
Altitude 230 m
Yellow fever: A yellow fever vaccination certificate is required from travellers over 1 year of age coming from infected areas.

Malaria: Malaria risk—predominantly due to *P. falciparum*—exists throughout the year in the whole country. Resistance to chloroquine reported.

Recommended prophylaxis: MEF.

GUINEA-BISSAU

Capital Bissau
Altitude 0 m
Yellow fever: A yellow fever vaccination certificate is required from travellers over 1 year of age coming from infected areas, and from the following countries:

Africa: Angola, Benin, Burkina Faso, Burundi, Cape Verde, Central African Republic, Chad, Congo, Côte d'Ivoire, Democratic Republic of the Congo, Djibouti, Equatorial Guinea, Ethiopia, Gabon, Gambia, Ghana, Guinea, Kenya, Liberia, Madagascar, Mali, Mauritania, Mozambique, Niger, Nigeria, Rwanda, Sao Tome and Principe, Senegal, Sierra Leone, Somalia, Togo, Uganda, United Republic of Tanzania, Zambia.

America: Bolivia, Brazil, Colombia, Ecuador, French Guiana, Guyana, Panama, Peru, Suriname, Venezuela.

Malaria: Malaria risk—predominantly due to *P. falciparum*—exists throughout the year in the whole country. Resistance to chloroquine reported.

Recommended prophylaxis: MEF.

GUYANA

Capital Georgetown

Altitude 0 m

Yellow fever: A yellow fever vaccination certificate is required from travellers coming from infected areas and from the following countries:

Africa: Angola, Benin, Burkina Faso, Burundi, Cameroon, Central African Republic, Chad, Congo, Côte d'Ivoire, Democratic Republic of the Congo, Gabon, Gambia, Ghana, Guinea, Guinea-Bissau, Kenya, Liberia, Mali, Niger, Nigeria, Rwanda, Sao Tome and Principe, Senegal, Sierra Leone, Somalia, Togo, Uganda, United Republic of Tanzania.

America: Belize, Bolivia, Brazil, Colombia, Costa Rica, Ecuador, French Guiana, Guatemala, Honduras, Nicaragua, Panama, Peru, Suriname, Venezuela.

Malaria: Malaria risk—*P. falciparum* (51%), *P. vivax* (49%)—is high throughout the year in all parts of the interior. Sporadic cases of malaria have been reported from the densely populated coastal belt. Chloroquine-resistant *P. falciparum* reported.

Recommended prophylaxis in risk areas: MEF.

HAITI

Capital Port-au-Prince

Altitude 100 m

Yellow fever: A yellow fever vaccination certificate is required from travellers coming from infected areas.

Malaria: Malaria risk—exclusively due to *P. falciparum*—exists throughout the year in certain forest areas in Chantal, Gros Morne, Hinche, Jacmel and Maissade. In the other cantons, risk is estimated to be low. No *P. falciparum* resistance to chloroquine reported.

Recommended prophylaxis in risk areas: CHL.

HONDURAS

Capital Tegucigalpa

Altitude 960 m

Yellow fever: A yellow fever vaccination certificate is required from travellers coming from infected areas.

Malaria: Malaria risk—predominantly due to *P. vivax*—is high throughout the year in 223 municipalities. Transmission risk is low in the other 71 municipalities, including San Pedro Sula and the city of Tegucigalpa. *P. falciparum* risk is the highest in Sanitary Region VI, including in the Islas de la Bahía.

Recommended prophylaxis : CHL.

HONG KONG SPECIAL ADMINISTRATIVE REGION OF CHINA *see* CHINA

HUNGARY

Capital Budapest

Altitude 110 m

No vaccination requirements for any international traveller.

ICELAND

Capital Reykjavik

Altitude 20 m

No vaccination requirements for any international traveller.

INDIA

Capital New Delhi

Altitude 210 m

Yellow fever: Anyone (except infants up to the age of 6 months) arriving by air or sea without a certificate is detained in isolation for up to 6 days if that person (*i*) arrives within 6 days of departure from an infected area, or (*ii*) has been in such an area in transit (excepting those passengers and members of the crew who, while in transit through an airport situated in an infected area, remained within the airport premises during the period of their entire stay and the Health Officer agrees to such exemption), or (*iii*) has come on a ship that started from or touched at any port in a yellow fever infected area up to 30 days before its arrival in India, unless such a ship has been disinsected in accordance with the procedure laid down by WHO, or (*iv*) has come by an aircraft which has been in an infected area and has not been disinsected in accordance with the provisions laid down in the Indian Aircraft Public Health Rules, 1954, or those recommended by WHO. The following countries and areas are regarded as infected:

Africa: Angola, Benin, Burkina Faso, Burundi, Cameroon, Central African Republic, Chad, Congo, Côte d'Ivoire, Democratic Republic of the Congo, Equatorial Guinea, Ethiopia, Gabon, Gambia, Ghana, Guinea, Guinea-Bissau, Kenya, Liberia, Mali, Niger, Nigeria, Rwanda, Sao Tome and Principe, Senegal, Sierra Leone, Somalia, Sudan, Togo, Uganda, United Republic of Tanzania, Zambia.

America: Bolivia, Brazil, Colombia, Ecuador, French Guiana, Guyana, Panama, Peru, Suriname, Trinidad and Tobago, Venezuela.

Note. When a case of yellow fever is reported from any country, that country is regarded by the Government of India as infected with yellow fever and is added to the above list.

Malaria: Malaria risk exists throughout the year in the whole country below 2000 m. There is no transmission in parts of the states of Himachal Pradesh, Jammu and Kashmir, and Sikkim. *P. falciparum* resistant to chloroquine and sulfadoxine–pyrimethamine reported.

Recommended prophylaxis: C+P.

INDONESIA

Capital Jakarta

Altitude 10 m

Yellow fever: A yellow fever vaccination certificate is required from travellers coming from infected areas. The countries and areas included in the endemic zones (see map page 84) are considered by Indonesia as infected areas.

Malaria: Malaria risk exists throughout the year in the whole country except in Jakarta Municipality, big cities, and the tourist resorts of Bali and Java. *P. falciparum* resistant to chloroquine and sulfadoxine–pyrimethamine reported. *P. vivax* resistant to chloroquine reported.

Recommended prophylaxis in risk areas: C+P; in Irian Jaya, MEF.

IRAN, ISLAMIC REPUBLIC OF

Capital Tehran

Altitude 1150 m

No vaccination requirements for any international traveller.

Malaria: Limited risk—exclusively due to *P. vivax*—exists in some areas north of the Zagros mountains and in western and south-western regions during the summer months. Malaria risk due to *P. falciparum* exists from March through November in rural areas of the provinces of Hormozgan, Kerman (tropical part) and Sistan–Baluchestan. *P. falciparum* resistant to chloroquine and sulfadoxine–pyrimethamine reported.

Recommended prophylaxis: CHL in *P. vivax* risk areas; C+P in *P. falciparum* risk areas.

IRAQ

Capital Baghdad

Altitude 40 m

Yellow fever: A yellow fever vaccination certificate is required from travellers coming from infected areas.

Malaria: Malaria risk—exclusively due to *P. vivax*—exists from May through November, principally in areas in the north below 1500 m (Duhok, Erbil, Ninawa, Sulaimaniya and Ta'mim provinces) but also in Basrah Province.

Recommended prophylaxis: CHL.

IRELAND

Capital Dublin

Altitude 30 m

No vaccination requirements for any international traveller.

ISRAEL

Capital Tel Aviv

Altitude 20 m

No vaccination requirements for any international traveller.

ITALY

Capital Rome

Altitude 30 m

No vaccination requirements for any international traveller.

JAMAICA

Capital Kingston

Altitude 30 m

Yellow fever: A yellow fever vaccination certificate is required from travellers over 1 year of age coming from infected areas.

JAPAN

Capital Tokyo

Altitude 10 m

No vaccination requirements for any international traveller.

JORDAN

Capital Amman

Altitude 800 m

Yellow fever: A yellow fever vaccination certificate is required from travellers over 1 year of age coming from infected areas.

KAZAKHSTAN

Capital Almaty

Altitude 860 m

Yellow fever: A yellow fever vaccination certificate is required from travellers coming from infected areas.

KENYA

Capital Nairobi

Altitude 1800 m

Yellow fever: A yellow fever vaccination certificate is required from travellers over 1 year of age coming from infected areas.

Malaria: Malaria risk—predominantly due to *P. falciparum*—exists throughout the year in the whole country. There is normally little risk in the city of Nairobi and in the highlands (above 2500 m) of Central, Eastern, Nyanza, Rift Valley and Western provinces. *P. falciparum* resistant to chloroquine and sulfadoxine–pyrimethamine reported.

Recommended prophylaxis: MEF.

KIRIBATI

Capital Tarawa

Altitude 0 m

Yellow fever: A yellow fever vaccination certificate is required from travellers over 1 year of age coming from infected areas.

KOREA, DEMOCRATIC PEOPLE'S REPUBLIC OF

Capital Pyongyang

Altitude 0 m

No vaccination requirements for any international traveller.

Malaria: Limited malaria risk—exclusively due to *P. vivax*—exists in some southern areas.

Recommended prophylaxis: none.

KOREA, REPUBLIC OF

Capital Seoul

Altitude 60 m

No vaccination requirements for any international traveller.

Malaria: Limited malaria risk—exclusively due to *P. vivax*—exists mainly in the northern areas of Kyunggi Do Province.

Recommended prophylaxis: none.

KUWAIT

Capital Kuwait

Altitude 30 m

No vaccination requirements for any international traveller.

KYRGYZSTAN

Capital Bishkek

Altitude 730 m

No vaccination requirements for any international traveller.

LAO PEOPLE'S DEMOCRATIC REPUBLIC

Capital Vientiane

Altitude 160 m

Yellow fever: A yellow fever vaccination certificate is required from travellers coming from infected areas.

Malaria: Malaria risk—predominantly due to *P. falciparum*—exists throughout the year in the whole country except in Vientiane. Chloroquine-resistant *P. falciparum* reported.

Recommended prophylaxis: MEF.

LATVIA

Capital Riga

Altitude 0 m

No vaccination requirements for any international traveller.

LEBANON

Capital Beirut
Altitude 50 m
Yellow fever: A yellow fever vaccination certificate is required from travellers coming from infected areas.

LESOTHO

Capital Maseru
Altitude 1700 m
Yellow fever: A yellow fever vaccination certificate is required from travellers coming from infected areas.

LIBERIA

Capital Monrovia
Altitude 10 m
Yellow fever: A yellow fever vaccination certificate is required from all travellers over 1 year of age.

Malaria: Malaria risk—predominantly due to *P. falciparum*—exists throughout the year in the whole country. *P. falciparum* resistant to chloroquine and sulfadoxine–pyrimethamine reported.

Recommended prophylaxis: MEF.

LIBYAN ARAB JAMAHIRIYA

Capital Tripoli
Altitude 20 m
Yellow fever: A yellow fever vaccination certificate is required from travellers coming from infected areas.

LIECHTENSTEIN

Capital Vaduz
Altitude 600 m
No vaccination requirements for any international traveller.

LITHUANIA

Capital Vilnius
Altitude 180 m
No vaccination requirements for any international traveller.

LUXEMBOURG

Capital Luxembourg
Altitude 340 m
No vaccination requirements for any international traveller.

MACAO SPECIAL ADMINISTRATIVE REGION OF CHINA *see* CHINA

MACEDONIA, THE FORMER YUGOSLAV REPUBLIC OF

Capital Skopje
Altitude 240 m
No vaccination requirements for any international traveller.

MADAGASCAR

Capital Antananarivo
Altitude 1300 m
Yellow fever: A yellow fever vaccination certificate is required from travellers coming from, or having been in transit in, areas considered to be infected.

Malaria: Malaria risk—predominantly due to *P. falciparum*—exists throughout the year in the whole country, with the highest risk in the coastal areas. Resistance to chloroquine reported.

Recommended prophylaxis: MEF.

MALAWI

Capital Lilongwe
Altitude 1030 m
Yellow fever: A yellow fever vaccination certificate is required from travellers coming from infected areas.

Malaria: Malaria risk—predominantly due to *P. falciparum*—exists throughout the year in the whole country. *P. falciparum* resistant to chloroquine and sulfadoxine–pyrimethamine reported.

Recommended prophylaxis: MEF.

MALAYSIA

Capital Kuala Lumpur
Altitude 50 m
Yellow fever: A yellow fever vaccination certificate is required from travellers over 1 year of age coming from infected areas. The countries and areas included in the endemic zones are considered as infected areas.

Malaria: Malaria risk exists only in limited foci in the deep hinterland. Urban and coastal areas are free from malaria, except in Sabah, where there is a risk—predominantly due to *P. falciparum*—throughout the year. *P. falciparum* resistant to chloroquine and sulfadoxine–pyrimethamine reported.

Recommended prophylaxis in risk areas: C+P; in Sabah, MEF.

MALDIVES

Capital Malé
Altitude 0 m
Yellow fever: A yellow fever vaccination certificate is required from travellers coming from infected areas.

MALI

Capital Bamako
Altitude 340 m
Yellow fever: A yellow fever vaccination certificate is required from all travellers over 1 year of age.
Malaria: Malaria risk—predominantly due to *P. falciparum*—exists throughout the year in the whole country. Resistance to chloroquine and sulfadoxine–pyrimethamine reported.
Recommended prophylaxis: MEF.

MALTA

Capital Valletta
Altitude 0 m
Yellow fever: A yellow fever vaccination certificate is required from travellers over 9 months of age coming from infected areas. If indicated on epidemiological grounds, infants under 9 months of age are subject to isolation or surveillance if coming from an infected area.

MARSHALL ISLANDS

Capital Majuro
Altitude 0 m
No vaccination requirements for any international traveller.

MARTINIQUE

Capital Fort-de-France
Altitude 0 m
No vaccination requirements for any international traveller.

MAURITANIA

Capital Nouakchott
Altitude 10 m
Yellow fever: A yellow fever vaccination certificate is required from all travellers over 1 year of age, except those arriving from a non-infected area and staying less than 2 weeks in the country.
Malaria: Malaria risk—predominantly due to *P. falciparum*—exists throughout the year in the whole country, except in the northern areas: Dakhlet-Nouadhibou and Tiris-Zemour. In Adrar and Inchiri there is malaria risk during the rainy season (July through October). Resistance to chloroquine reported.
Recommended prophylaxis in risk areas: C+P.

MAURITIUS

Capital Port Louis
Altitude 90 m
Yellow fever: A yellow fever vaccination certificate is required from travellers over 1 year of age coming from infected areas. The countries and areas included in the endemic zones (see map page 84) are considered as infected areas.
Malaria: Malaria risk—exclusively due to *P. vivax*—exists in certain rural areas. There is no risk on Rodrigues Island.
Recommended prophylaxis: none.

MAYOTTE (FRENCH TERRITORIAL COLLECTIVITY)

Capital Mamoudzou
Altitude 280 m
No vaccination requirements for any international traveller.
Malaria: Malaria risk—predominantly due to *P. falciparum*—exists throughout the year.
Recommended prophylaxis: MEF.

MEXICO

Capital Mexico City
Altitude 2250 m
Yellow fever: No vaccination requirements for any international traveller.
Malaria: Malaria risk—almost exclusively due to *P. vivax*—exists throughout the year in some rural areas that are not often visited by tourists. There is high risk of transmission in some localities in the states of Chiapas, Quintana Roo, Sinaloa and Tabasco; moderate risk in the states of Chihuahua, Durango, Nayarit, Oaxaca and Sonora; and low risk in Campeche, Guerrero, Michoacán and Jalisco.
Recommended prophylaxis in risk areas: CHL.

MICRONESIA, FEDERATED STATES OF

Capital Palikir

Altitude 0 m

No vaccination requirements for any international traveller.

MOLDOVA, REPUBLIC OF

Capital Chisinau

Altitude 100 m

No vaccination requirements for any international traveller.

MONACO

Capital Monaco

Altitude 0 m

No vaccination requirements for any international traveller.

MONGOLIA

Capital Ulaanbaatar

Altitude 1300 m

No vaccination requirements for any international traveller.

MONTSERRAT

Capital Plymouth

Altitude 120 m

No vaccination requirements for any international traveller.

MOROCCO

Capital Rabat

Altitude 0 m

No vaccination requirements for any international traveller.

Malaria: Very limited malaria risk—exclusively due to *P. vivax*—may exist from May to October in certain rural areas of Khourigba Province. Risk for travellers in such areas extremely low.

Recommended prophylaxis: none.

MOZAMBIQUE

Capital Maputo

Altitude 50 m

Yellow fever: A yellow fever vaccination certificate is required from travellers over 1 year of age coming from infected areas.

Malaria: Malaria risk—predominantly due to *P. falciparum*—exists throughout the year in the whole country. *P. falciparum* resistant to chloroquine and sulfadoxine–pyrimethamine reported.

Recommended prophylaxis: MEF.

MYANMAR (FORMERLY BURMA)

Capital Yangon

Altitude 20 m

Yellow fever: A yellow fever vaccination certificate is required from travellers coming from infected areas. Nationals and residents of Myanmar are required to possess certificates of vaccination on their departure to an infected area.

Malaria: Malaria risk—predominantly due to *P. falciparum*—exists commonly below 1000 m *(a)* throughout the year in Karen State; *(b)* from March through December in Chin, Kachin, Kayah, Mon, Rakhine and Shan states, Pegu Division, and Hlegu, Hmawbi, and Taikkyi townships of Yangon (formerly Rangoon) Division; *(c)* from April through December in the rural areas of Tenasserim Division; *(d)* from May through December in Irrawaddy Division and the rural areas of Mandalay Division; *(e)* from June through November in the rural areas of Magwe Division, and in Sagaing Division. *P. falciparum* resistant to chloroquine and sulfadoxine–pyrimethamine reported. Mefloquine resistance reported in the eastern part of Shan State. *P. vivax* resistant to chloroquine reported.

Recommended prophylaxis: MEF; in eastern part of Shan State, DOX.

NAMIBIA

Capital Windhoek

Altitude 1720 m

Yellow fever: A yellow fever vaccination certificate is required from travellers coming from infected areas. The countries, or parts of countries, included in the endemic zones in Africa and South America are regarded as infected,

Travellers on scheduled flights that originated outside the areas regarded as infected, but who have been in transit through these areas, are not required to possess a certificate provided that they remained at the scheduled airport or in the adjacent town during transit. All passengers whose flights originated in infected areas or who have been in transit through these areas on unscheduled flights are required to possess a certificate. The certificate is not insisted upon in the case of children under 1 year of age, but such infants may be subject to surveillance.

Malaria: Malaria risk—predominantly due to *P. falciparum*—exists from November to May/June in the northern regions and in Omaheke and Otjozondjupa and throughout the year along the Kavango and Kunene rivers. Resistance to chloroquine reported.

Recommended prophylaxis in risk areas: C+P.

NAURU

Capital Yaren

Altitude 10 m

Yellow fever: A yellow fever vaccination certificate is required from travellers over 1 year of age coming from infected areas.

NEPAL

Capital Kathmandu

Altitude 1300 m

Yellow fever: A yellow fever vaccination certificate is required from travellers coming from infected areas.

Malaria: Malaria risk—predominantly due to *P. vivax*—exists throughout the year in rural areas of the Terai districts (including forested hills and forest areas) of Bara, Dhanukha, Kapilvastu, Mahotari, Parsa, Rautahat, Rupendehi and Sarlahi, and especially along the Indian border. *P. falciparum* resistant to chloroquine and sulfadoxine–pyrimethamine reported.

Recommended prophylaxis in risk areas: C+P.

NETHERLANDS

Capital Amsterdam / The Hague
(seat of Government)

Altitude 0 m / 0 m

No vaccination requirements for any international traveller.

NETHERLANDS ANTILLES

Capital Willemstad

Altitude 0 m

Yellow fever: A yellow fever vaccination certificate is required from travellers over 6 months of age coming from infected area

NEW CALEDONIA AND DEPENDENCIES

Capital Nouméa

Altitude 10 m

Cholera: Vaccination against cholera is not required. Travellers coming from an infected area

are not given chemoprophylaxis, but are required to complete a form for use by the Health Service.

Yellow fever: A yellow fever vaccination certificate is required from travellers over 1 year of age coming from infected areas.

Note. In the event of an epidemic threat to the territory, a specific vaccination certificate may be required.

NEW ZEALAND

Capital Wellington

Altitude 70 m

No vaccination requirements for any international traveller.

NICARAGUA

Capital Managua

Altitude 70 m

Yellow fever: A yellow fever vaccination certificate is required from travellers over 1 year of age coming from infected areas.

Malaria: Malaria risk—predominantly due to *P. vivax*—is high throughout the year in 119 municipalities, with the highest risk in Chinandega, Jinotega, Nueva Segovía, RAAN, RAAS and Rio San Juan. In the other 26 municipalities, in the departments of Carazo, Madriz and Masaya, transmission risk is low or negligible. No chloroquine-resistant *P. falciparum* reported.

Recommended prophylaxis in risk areas: CHL.

NIGER

Capital Niamey

Altitude 220 m

Yellow fever: A yellow fever vaccination certificate is required from all travellers over 1 year of age and recommended for travellers leaving Niger.

Malaria: Malaria risk—predominantly due to *P. falciparum*—exists throughout the year in the whole country. Chloroquine-resistant *P. falciparum* reported.

Recommended prophylaxis: MEF.

NIGERIA

Capital Abuja

Altitude 360 m

Yellow fever: A yellow fever vaccination certificate is required from travellers over 1 year of age coming from infected areas.

Malaria: Malaria risk—predominantly due to *P. falciparum*—exists throughout the year in the whole country. *P. falciparum* resistant to chloroquine and sulfadoxine–pyrimethamine reported.

Recommended prophylaxis: MEF.

NIUE

Capital Alofi
Altitude 10 m
Yellow fever: A yellow fever vaccination certificate is required from travellers over 1 year of age coming from infected areas.

NORTHERN MARIANA ISLANDS

Capital Saipan
Altitude 0 m
No vaccination requirements for any international traveller.

NORWAY

Capital Oslo
Altitude 50 m
No vaccination requirements for any international traveller.

OMAN

Capital Muscat
Altitude 20 m
Yellow fever: A yellow fever vaccination certificate is required from travellers coming from infected areas.

Malaria: Very limited malaria risk—including *P. falciparum*—may exist in remote areas of Musandam Province. Chloroquine-resistant *P. falciparum* reported. Risk for travellers in such areas extremely low.

Recommended prophylaxis : none.

PAKISTAN

Capital Islamabad
Altitude 350 m
Yellow fever: A yellow fever vaccination certificate is required from travellers coming from any part of a country in which yellow fever is endemic; infants under 6 months of age are exempt if the mother's vaccination certificate shows that she was vaccinated before the birth of the child. The

countries and areas included in the endemic zones are considered as infected areas.

Malaria: Malaria risk exists throughout the year in the whole country below 2000 m. *P. falciparum* resistant to chloroquine and sulfadoxine–pyrimethamine reported.

Recommended prophylaxis: C+P.

PALAU

Capital Koror
Altitude 0 m
Yellow fever: A yellow fever vaccination certificate is required from all travellers over 1 year of age coming from infected areas or from countries in any part of which yellow fever is endemic.

PANAMA

Capital Panama City
Altitude 20 m
Yellow fever: A yellow fever vaccination certificate is recommended for all travellers going to Chepo, Darién and San Blas.

Malaria: Low malaria risk—predominantly due to *P. vivax*—occurs throughout the year in three provinces: Bocas del Toro in the west and Darién and San Blas in the east. In the other provinces there is no or negligible risk of transmission. Chloroquine-resistant *P. falciparum* has been reported in Darién and San Blas provinces.

Recommended prophylaxis in risk areas: CHL; in eastern endemic areas, MEF.

PAPUA NEW GUINEA

Capital Port Moresby
Altitude 20 m
Yellow fever: A yellow fever vaccination certificate is required from all travellers over 1 year of age coming from infected areas.

Malaria: Malaria risk—predominantly due to *P. falciparum*—exists throughout the year in the whole country below 1800 m. *P. falciparum* resistant to chloroquine and sulfadoxine–pyrimethamine reported. *P. vivax* resistant to chloroquine reported.

Recommended prophylaxis: MEF.

PARAGUAY

Capital Asunción
Altitude 60 m

Yellow fever: A yellow fever vaccination certificate is required from travellers leaving Paraguay to go to endemic areas and from travellers coming from endemic areas.

Malaria: Malaria risk—exclusively due to P. vivax—is moderate in certain municipalities of the departments of Alto Paraná, Caaguazú and Canendiyú. In the other 14 departments there is no or negligible transmission risk.

Recommended prophylaxis in risk areas: CHL.

PERU

Capital Lima
Altitude 90 m
Yellow fever: Yellow fever vaccination is required from travellers over 6 months of age coming from infected areas and is recommended for those who intend to visit jungle areas of the country below 2300 m.

Malaria: Malaria risk—P. vivax (69%), P. falciparum (31%)—is high in 21 of the 33 sanitary regions, including Ayacucho, Cajamarca, Cerro de Pasco, Chachapoyas, Chanca-Andahuaylas, Cutervo, Cusco, Huancavelica, Jaen, Junín, La Libertad, Lambayeque, Loreto, Madre de Dios, Piura, San Martín, Tumbes and Ucayali.

P. falciparum transmission reported in Jaen, Lambayeque, Loreto, Luciano Castillo, Piura, San Martín, Tumbes and Ucayali. Resistance to chloroquine and sulfadoxine–pyrimethamine reported.

Recommended prophylaxis: CHL in P. vivax risk areas; MEF in P. falciparum risk areas.

PHILIPPINES

Capital Manila
Altitude 20 m
Yellow fever: A yellow fever vaccination certificate is required from travellers over 1 year of age coming from infected areas.

Malaria: Malaria risk exists throughout the year in areas below 600 m, except in the provinces of Bohol, Catanduanes, Cebu, and metropolitan Manila. There is low risk in the provinces of Aklan, Biliran, Camiguin, Capiz, Guimaras, Iloilo, Leyte del Sur, Northern Samar and Sequijor. No risk is considered to exist in urban areas or in the plains. P. falciparum resistant to chloroquine and sulfadoxine–pyrimethamine reported.

Recommended prophylaxis in risk areas: C+P.

PITCAIRN

Capital Adamstown
Altitude 0 m
Yellow fever: A yellow fever vaccination certificate is required from travellers over 1 year of age coming from infected areas.

POLAND

Capital Warsaw
Altitude 100 m
No vaccination requirements for any international traveller.

PORTUGAL

Capital Lisbon
Altitude 50 m
Yellow fever: A yellow fever vaccination certificate is required from travellers over 1 year of age coming from infected areas. The requirement applies only to travellers arriving in or bound for the Azores and Madeira. However, no certificate is required from passengers in transit at Funchal, Porto Santo and Santa Maria.

PUERTO RICO

Capital San Juan
Altitude 10 m
No vaccination requirements for any international traveller.

QATAR

Capital Doha
Altitude 20 m
No vaccination requirements for any international traveller.

REUNION

Capital Saint-Denis
Altitude 0 m
Yellow fever: A yellow fever vaccination certificate is required from travellers over 1 year of age coming from infected areas.

ROMANIA

Capital Bucharest
Altitude 80 m
No vaccination requirements for any international traveller.

RUSSIAN FEDERATION

Capital Moscow
Altitude 160 m
No vaccination requirements for any international traveller.

RWANDA

Capital Kigali
Altitude 1550 m
Yellow fever: A yellow fever vaccination certificate is required from all travellers over 1 year of age.

Malaria: Malaria risk—predominantly due to *P. falciparum*—exists throughout the year in the whole country. *P. falciparum* resistant to chloroquine and sulfadoxine–pyrimethamine reported.

Recommended prophylaxis: MEF.

SAINT HELENA

Capital Jamestown
Altitude 0 m
Yellow fever: A yellow fever vaccination certificate is required from travellers over 1 year of age coming from infected areas.

SAINT KITTS AND NEVIS

Capital Basseterre
Altitude 360 m
Yellow fever: A yellow fever vaccination certificate is required from travellers over 1 year of age coming from infected areas.

SAINT LUCIA

Capital Castries
Altitude 200 m
Yellow fever: A yellow fever vaccination certificate is required from travellers over 1 year of age coming from infected areas

SAINT PIERRE AND MIQUELON

Capital Saint-Pierre
Altitude 360 m
No vaccination requirements for any international traveller.

SAINT VINCENT AND THE GRENADINES

Capital Kingstown
Altitude 0 m

Yellow fever: A yellow fever vaccination certificate is required from travellers over 1 year of age coming from infected areas.

SAMOA

Capital Apia
Altitude 0 m
Yellow fever: A yellow fever vaccination certificate is required from travellers over 1 year of age coming from infected areas.

SAN MARINO

Capital San Marino
Altitude 290 m
No vaccination requirements for any international traveller.

SAO TOME AND PRINCIPE

Capital Sao Tomé
Altitude 0 m
Yellow fever: A yellow fever vaccination certificate is required from all travellers over 1 year of age.

Malaria: Malaria risk—predominantly due to *P. falciparum*—exists throughout the year. Chloroquine-resistant *P. falciparum* reported.

Recommended prophylaxis: MEF.

SAUDI ARABIA

Capital Riyadh
Altitude 610 m
Yellow fever: A yellow fever vaccination certificate is required from all travellers coming from countries, any parts of which are infected.

Malaria: Malaria risk—predominantly due to *P. falciparum*—exists throughout the year in most of the Southern Region (except in the high-altitude areas of Asir Province) and in certain rural areas of the Western Region. No risk in Mecca or Medina. Chloroquine-resistant *P. falciparum* reported.

Recommended prophylaxis in risk areas: C+P.

SENEGAL

Capital Dakar
Altitude 20 m
Yellow fever: A yellow fever vaccination certificate is required from travellers coming from endemic areas.

Malaria: Malaria risk—predominantly due to *P. falciparum*—exists throughout the year in the whole country. There is less risk from January through June in the central western regions. Resistance to chloroquine and sulfadoxine–pyrimethamine reported.

Recommended prophylaxis: MEF.

SEYCHELLES

Capital Victoria

Altitude 0 m

Yellow fever: A yellow fever vaccination certificate is required from travellers over 1 year of age coming from infected areas or who have passed through partly or wholly endemic areas within the preceding 6 days. The countries and areas included in the endemic zones are considered as infected areas.

SIERRA LEONE

Capital Freetown

Altitude 50 m

Yellow fever: A yellow fever vaccination certificate is required from travellers coming from infected areas.

Malaria: Malaria risk—predominantly due to *P. falciparum*—exists throughout the year in the whole country. Resistance to chloroquine reported.

Recommended prophylaxis: MEF.

SINGAPORE

Capital Singapore

Altitude 50 m

Yellow fever: A yellow fever vaccination certificate is required from travellers over 1 year of age coming from infected areas. Certificates of vaccination are required from travellers over 1 year of age who, within the preceding 6 days, have been in or have passed through any country partly or wholly endemic for yellow fever. The countries and areas included in the endemic zones are considered as infected areas.

SLOVAKIA

Capital Bratislava

Altitude 130 m

No vaccination requirements for any international traveller.

SLOVENIA

Capital Ljubljana

Altitude 320 m

No vaccination requirements for any international traveller.

SOLOMON ISLANDS

Capital Honiara

Altitude 30 m

Yellow fever: A yellow fever vaccination certificate is required from travellers coming from infected areas.

Malaria: Malaria risk—predominantly due to *P. falciparum*—exists throughout the year except in a few eastern and southern outlying islets. *P. falciparum* resistant to chloroquine and sulfadoxine–pyrimethamine reported.

Recommended prophylaxis: C+P.

SOMALIA

Capital Mogadishu

Altitude 20 m

Yellow fever: A yellow fever vaccination certificate is required from travellers coming from infected areas.

Malaria: Malaria risk—predominantly due to *P. falciparum*—exists throughout the year in the whole country. Resistance to chloroquine and sulfadoxine–pyrimethamine reported.

Recommended prophylaxis: MEF.

SOUTH AFRICA

Capital Pretoria (administrative) / Cape Town (legislative) / Bloemfontein (judicial)

Altitude 1330 m / 10 m / 1420 m

Yellow fever: A yellow fever vaccination certificate is required from travellers over 1 year of age coming from infected areas. The countries or areas included in the endemic zones in Africa and the Americas are regarded as infected (see map page 84).

Malaria: Malaria risk—predominantly due to *P. falciparum*—exists throughout the year in the low altitude areas of Mpumalanga Province (including the Kruger National Park), Northern Province and north-eastern KwaZulu-Natal as far south as the Tugela River. Risk is highest from October to May. Resistance to chloroquine and sulfadoxine–pyrimethamine reported.

Recommended prophylaxis in risk areas: MEF.

SPAIN

Capital Madrid
Altitude 600 m
No vaccination requirements for any international traveller.

SRI LANKA

Capital Colombo
Altitude 10 m
Yellow fever: A yellow fever vaccination certificate is required from travellers over 1 year of age coming from infected areas.

Malaria: Malaria risk—predominantly due to *P. vivax*—exists throughout the year in the whole country excluding the districts of Colombo, Kalutara and Nuwara Eliya. *P. falciparum* resistant to chloroquine and sulfadoxine–pyrimethamine reported.

Recommended prophylaxis: C+P.

SUDAN

Capital Khartoum
Altitude 380 m
Yellow fever: A yellow fever vaccination certificate is required from travellers over 1 year of age coming from infected areas. The countries and areas included in the endemic zones (see map page 84) are considered as infected areas. A certificate may be required from travellers leaving Sudan.

Malaria: Malaria risk—predominantly due to *P. falciparum*—exists throughout the year in the whole country. Risk is low and seasonal in the north. It is higher along the Nile south of Lake Nasser and in the central and southern part of the country. Malaria risk on the Red Sea coast is very limited. *P. falciparum* resistant to chloroquine and sulfadoxine–pyrimethamine reported.

Recommended prophylaxis: MEF.

SURINAME

Capital Paramaribo
Altitude 0 m
Yellow fever: A yellow fever vaccination certificate is required from travellers coming from infected areas.

Malaria: Malaria risk—*P. falciparum* (86%), *P. vivax* (14%)—is high throughout the year in the three southern districts of the country. In Paramaribo city and the other seven coastal districts, transmission risk is low or negligible. *P. falciparum* resistant to chloroquine and sulfadoxine–pyrimethamine reported. Some decline in quinine sensitivity also reported.

Recommended prophylaxis in risk areas: MEF.

SWAZILAND

Capital Mbabane (administrative) /
Lolamba (legislative)
Altitude 1240 m / 650 m
Yellow fever: A yellow fever vaccination certificate is required from travellers coming from infected areas.

Malaria: Malaria risk—predominantly due to *P. falciparum*—exists throughout the year in all low veld areas (mainly Big Bend, Mhlume, Simunye and Tshaneni). Chloroquine-resistant *P. falciparum* reported.

Recommended prophylaxis in risk areas: MEF.

SWEDEN

Capital Stockholm
Altitude 30 m
No vaccination requirements for any international traveller.

SWITZERLAND

Capital Berne
Altitude 520 m
No vaccination requirements for any international traveller.

SYRIAN ARAB REPUBLIC

Capital Damascus
Altitude 700 m
Yellow fever: A yellow fever vaccination certificate is required from travellers coming from infected areas.

Malaria: Malaria risk—exclusively due to *P. vivax*—exists from May through October in foci along the northern border, especially in the north-eastern part of the country.

Recommended prophylaxis in risk areas: CHL.

TAJIKISTAN

Capital Dushanbe
Altitude 1030 m

No vaccination requirements for any international traveller.

Malaria: Malaria risk—predominantly due to *P. vivax*—exists from June through October, particularly in southern border areas (Khatlon Region), and in some central (Dushanbe), western (Gorno-Badakhshan), and northern (Leninabad Region) areas. Chloroquine-resistant *P. falciparum* suspected in some areas.

Recommended prophylaxis in risk areas: CHL.

TANZANIA, UNITED REPUBLIC OF

Capital Dodoma

Altitude 1150 m

Yellow fever: A yellow fever vaccination certificate is required from travellers over 1 year of age coming from infected areas. The countries and areas included in the endemic zones are considered as infected areas.

Malaria: Malaria risk—predominantly due to *P. falciparum*—exists throughout the year in the whole country below 1800 m. *P. falciparum* resistant to chloroquine and sulfadoxine–pyrimethamine reported.

Recommended prophylaxis: MEF.

THAILAND

Capital Bangkok

Altitude 10 m

Yellow fever: A yellow fever vaccination certificate is required from travellers over 1 year of age coming from infected areas. The countries and areas included in the endemic zones are considered as infected areas.

Malaria: Malaria risk exists throughout the year in rural, especially forested and hilly, areas of the whole country, mainly towards the international borders. There is no risk in cities and the main tourist resorts (e.g. Bangkok, Chiangmai, Pattaya, Phuket, Samui). *P. falciparum* resistant to chloroquine and sulfadoxine–pyrimethamine reported. Resistance to mefloquine and to quinine reported from areas near the borders with Cambodia and Myanmar.

Recommended prophylaxis in risk areas near Cambodia and Myanmar borders: DOX.

TOGO

Capital Lomé

Altitude 40 m

Yellow fever: A yellow fever vaccination certificate is required from all travellers over 1 year of age.

Malaria: Malaria risk—predominantly due to *P. falciparum*—exists throughout the year in the whole country. Chloroquine-resistant *P. falciparum* reported.

Recommended prophylaxis: MEF.

TOKELAU

Same requirements as New Zealand.

(Non-self governing territory of New Zealand)

TONGA

Capital Nuku'alofa

Altitude 0 m

Yellow fever: A yellow fever vaccination certificate is required from travellers over 1 year of age coming from infected areas.

TRINIDAD AND TOBAGO

Capital Port of Spain

Altitude 10 m

Yellow fever: A yellow fever vaccination certificate is required from travellers over 1 year of age coming from infected areas.

TUNISIA

Capital Tunis

Altitude 50 m

Yellow fever: A yellow fever vaccination certificate is required from travellers over 1 year of age coming from infected areas.

TURKEY

Capital Ankara

Altitude 920 m

No vaccination requirements for any international traveller.

Malaria: Malaria risk—exclusively due to *P. vivax*—exists from May to October mainly in the south-eastern part of the country, and in Amikova and Çukurova Plain. There is no malaria risk in the main tourist areas in the west and south-west of the country.

Recommended prophylaxis in risk areas: CHL.

TURKMENISTAN

Capital Ashkabat

Altitude 220 m

No vaccination requirements for any international traveller.

Malaria: Malaria risk—exclusively due to *P. vivax*—exists from June to October in some villages located in the south-eastern part of the country, mainly in Mary district.

Recommended prophylaxis: none.

TUVALU

Capital Fongafale

Altitude 0 m

No vaccination requirements for any international traveller.

UGANDA

Capital Kampala

Altitude 1200 m

Yellow fever: A yellow fever vaccination certificate is required from travellers over 1 year of age coming from endemic areas.

Malaria: Malaria risk—predominantly due to *P. falciparum*—exists throughout the year in the whole country including the main towns of Fort Portal, Jinja, Kampala, Mbale and parts of Kigezi. Resistance to chloroquine and sulfadoxine–pyrimethamine reported.

Recommended prophylaxis: MEF.

UKRAINE

Capital Kiev

Altitude 170 m

No vaccination requirements for any international traveller.

UNITED ARAB EMIRATES

Capital Abu Dhabi

Altitude 10 m

No vaccination requirements for any international traveller.

Malaria: Very limited malaria risk in the foothill areas and valleys in the mountainous regions of the northern Emirates bordering Oman Musandam Province.

Recommended prophylaxis: none.

UNITED KINGDOM (with Channel Islands and Isle of Man)

Capital London

Altitude 10 m

No vaccination requirements for any international traveller.

UNITED STATES OF AMERICA

Capital Washington DC

Altitude 20 m

No vaccination requirements for any international traveller.

URUGUAY

Capital Montevideo

Altitude 30 m

No vaccination requirements for any international traveller.

UZBEKISTAN

Capital Tashkent

Altitude 460 m

No vaccination requirements for any international traveller.

Malaria: Sporadic autochthonous cases of *P. vivax* malaria are reported from Surkhandarinskaya Region (Uzunskiy, Sariassiskiy and Shurchinskiy districts).

Recommended prophylaxis: none.

VANUATU

Capital Port-Vila

Altitude 0 m

No vaccination requirements for any international traveller.

Malaria: Low to moderate malaria risk—predominantly due to *P. falciparum*—exists throughout the year in the whole country. *P. falciparum* resistant to chloroquine and sulfadoxine–pyrimethamine reported. *P. vivax* resistant to chloroquine reported.

Recommended prophylaxis: C+P.

VENEZUELA

Capital Caracas

Altitude 1000 m

No vaccination requirements for any international traveller.

Malaria: Malaria risk due to *P. vivax* exists throughout the year in some rural areas of Apure, Amazonas, Barinas, Bolívar, Sucre and Táchira states. Risk of *P. falciparum* malaria is restricted to municipalities in jungle areas of Amazonas (Atabapo), Bolívar (Cedeño, Gran Sabana, Raul Leoni, Sifontes and Sucre) and Delta Amacuro (Antonia Diaz, Casacoima and Pedernales). Chloroquine-resistant *P. falciparum* confirmed in the interior of Amazonas state.

Recommended prophylaxis: CHL in *P. vivax* risk areas; MEF in *P. falciparum* risk areas.

VIET NAM

Capital Hanoi

Altitude 20 m

Yellow fever: A yellow fever vaccination certificate is required from travellers over 1 year of age coming from infected areas.

Malaria: Malaria risk exists in the whole country, excluding urban centres, the Red River delta, and the coastal plains north of Nha Trang. High-risk areas are the two southernmost provinces of the country, Ca Mau and Bac Lieu, and the highland areas below 1500 m south of 18°N. Most cases are caused by *P. falciparum*, which in most areas is resistant to chloroquine and sulfadoxine–pyrimethamine.

Recommended prophylaxis: MEF.

VIRGIN ISLANDS (USA)

Capital Charlotte Amalie

Altitude 230 m

No vaccination requirements for any international traveller.

WAKE ISLAND

No vaccination requirements for any international traveller.

(US territory)

YEMEN

Capital Sana'a

Altitude 2230 m

Yellow fever: A yellow fever vaccination certificate is required from travellers over 1 year of age coming from infected areas.

Malaria: Malaria risk—predominantly due to *P. falciparum*—exists throughout the year, but mainly from September through February, in the whole country below 2000 m. There is no risk in Sana'a. Resistance to chloroquine reported.

Recommended prophylaxis: C+P.

YUGOSLAVIA, FEDERAL REPUBLIC OF

Capital Belgrade

Altitude 60 m

No vaccination requirements for any international traveller.

ZAIRE *see* CONGO, DEMOCRATIC REPUBLIC OF THE

ZAMBIA

Capital Lusaka

Altitude 1280 m

Yellow fever: No vaccination requirements for any international traveller.

Malaria: Malaria risk—predominantly due to *P. falciparum*—exists throughout the year in the whole country. Resistance to chloroquine and sulfadoxine–pyrimethamine reported.

Recommended prophylaxis: MEF.

ZIMBABWE

Capital Harare

Altitude 1450 m

Yellow fever: A yellow fever vaccination certificate is required from travellers coming from infected areas.

Malaria: Malaria risk—predominantly due to *P. falciparum*—exists from November through June in areas below 1200 m and throughout the year in the Zambezi valley. In Harare and Bulawayo, the risk is negligible. Resistance to chloroquine reported.

Recommended prophylaxis: MEF.

Approved yellow fever vaccine producers

Manufacturers or agency	Address of manufacturer or distributor
Aventis Pasteur, France	58, avenue Leclerc BP 7046 69348 Lyon Cedex 07 France
BioManguinhos, Brazil	Av Brasil 4365 – Manguinhos 21045-900 Rio de Janeiro/RJ Brazil
Institut Pasteur Dakar, Senegal	BP 220 36, avenue Pasteur Dakar Senegal
Celltech Group plc, (formerly Medeva, U.K.)	Evans House, Regent Park Kingston Road Leatherhead LT22 7PQ United Kingdom

International Health Regulations

The globalization of infectious diseases is not a new phenomenon. However, increased population movements, whether through tourism or migration or as a result of disasters; growth in international trade in food and biological products; social and environmental changes linked with urbanization, deforestation and alterations in climate; and changes in methods of food processing, distribution and consumer habits have reaffirmed that infectious disease events in one country are potentially a concern for the entire world. In addition to epidemics that occur naturally, outbreaks might result from intentional or accidental release of biological agents. Consequently, the need for international cooperation in order to safeguard global health security is as crucial as ever.

The International Health Regulations, adopted in 1969 and amended in 1973 and 1981,[1] provide the framework for such international cooperation. Their stated purpose is "to ensure maximum security against international spread of diseases with minimum interference with world traffic and trade". Their main objectives are to ensure: (1) the consistent application of routine, preventive measures (e.g. at ports and airports) and the use by all of internationally approved documents (e.g. vaccination certificates); and (2) the formal notification to WHO and implementation of predetermined measures in the event of the occurrence of one of the three notifiable diseases (cholera, plague and yellow fever). The two main practical applications of the Regulations likely to be encountered by travellers are the yellow fever vaccination requirements imposed by certain countries (see Chapter 6 and page 151) and the disinsection of aircraft to prevent importation of disease vectors (see Chapter 2).

These measures are intended to help prevent the international spread of diseases and, in the context of international travel, to do so with the minimum inconvenience to the passenger. This requires international collaboration in the detection and reduction or elimination of the sources from which infection

---

[1] *International Health Regulations (1969): third annotated edition*. Geneva, World Health Organization, 1983.

spreads rather than attempts to prevent the introduction of disease by legalistic barriers that over the years have proved to be ineffective. Ultimately, however, the risk of an infective agent becoming established in a country is determined by the quality of the national epidemiological services and, in particular, by day-to-day national health and disease surveillance activities and the ability to implement prompt and effective control measures.

The International Health Regulations are currently being revised, in order to ensure that they are better adapted to the present volume of international traffic and trade and take account of current trends in the epidemiology of infectious diseases, including emerging disease threats. The main proposed shift is to depart from the three diseases mentioned above and to focus on any "health emergency of international concern". The main challenges encountered during the revision include: ensuring that only public health risks (usually caused by an infectious agent) that are of urgent international importance are reported under the Regulations; avoiding stigmatization and unnecessary negative impact on international travel and trade of invalid reporting from sources other than Member States, which can have serious economic consequences for countries; and making sure that the system is sensitive enough to detect new or re-emerging public health risks.

Index of countries and territories

Index by subject